Cat Care

A Guide for Pet Lovers

Cat Care

A Guide for Pet Lovers

by
Dr. Geeta
M.V.Sc. (Surgery), MBA

2011
DAYA PUBLISHING HOUSE
Delhi - 110 002

© 2011, GEETA (b. 1977–   )
ISBN 9788170359821

Published by	:	**Daya Publishing House** **A Division of** **Astral International Pvt. Ltd.** **– ISO 9001:2008 Certified Company –** 4760-61/23, Ansari Road, Darya Ganj, New Delhi - 110 002 Phone: 23245578, 23244987 Fax: (011) 23260116 e-mail : dayabooks@vsnl.com website : www.dayabooks.com
Laser Typesetting	:	**Classic Computer Services** Delhi - 110 035
Printed at	:	**Chawla Offset Printers** Delhi - 110 052

PRINTED IN INDIA

for

Danny and Yadavi

Preface

This book is basically a practical guide for the owners, veterinary students and is a reference book for the practicing Veterinary surgeons. I have put my best knowledge and practical experiences for the readers to help them to understand the nature of pet, different issues related to their health and day to day problems experienced by the owners due to lack of knowledge.

This indispensable book will tell you everything you need to know about the care, feeding and training of your cat. Details have been provided about the kitten or cat examination, signs of ill or good health. This book comprises a chapter about how to prevent clawing of furniture, care of older cat, general care and grooming, behaviour, and introduction of new kitten or cat to your home. Detailed information has been provided about handling, grooming, neutering and breeding.

Complete information has been provided about hoe to take care of an orphan kitten, first aid for an injured cat. An alternate approach delves into the fascinating world of complementary treatment ranging from acupuncture, homoeopathy, herbal medicines, acupressure and physiotherapy.

This book is the essential guide for anyone who has a cat or planning to adopt one. Photographs illustrate subjects like socialization, handling, grooming, house breaking and prevention of behaviour problems. It contains all the information to keep a kitten happy, healthy and in top condition.

Dr. Geeta

Contents

Preface   *vii*

1. Introduction   1

2. Source to Look for a Cat   7

3. How to Choose your Kitten: Personality
   and Health   14

4. Kitten   20

5. Kitten Supplies   28

6. Bringing Home a New Cat or Kitten   35

7. Selecting a Name for your Kitten   41

8. Litter Box Training   43

9. Kitten Proofing your Home   48

10. Car Sickness   51

11. Administering Medicines   53

12. Care of Coat   59

13. Care of Eyes — 66

14. Care of Ear — 68

15. Dental Care — 73

16. Hairballs — 77

17. Clipping Nails — 79

18. Feeding — 82

19. Anatomy of a Cat — 88

20. Going on Vacation — 95

21. Traveling and Shipping — 100

22. Understanding your Cat — 108

23. Vaccination — 115

24. Pet Health Insurance — 121

25. Name Tags — 123

26. How to Choose the Right Veterinarian — 124

27. Annual Veterinary Exams — 126

28. Care of Older Cats — 128

29. Breeding — 139

30. Spaying — 151

31. Some Myths — 155

32. Health Care — 157

33. First Aid — 168

34. Cat Horoscope — 172

35. Alternative Therapy — 180

36. Cat Breeds — 185

Index — 189

1
Introduction

Some people have owned cats all their lives and they feel that home is incomplete without a resident cat. While for others, owning a cat is a pleasure discovered later in life

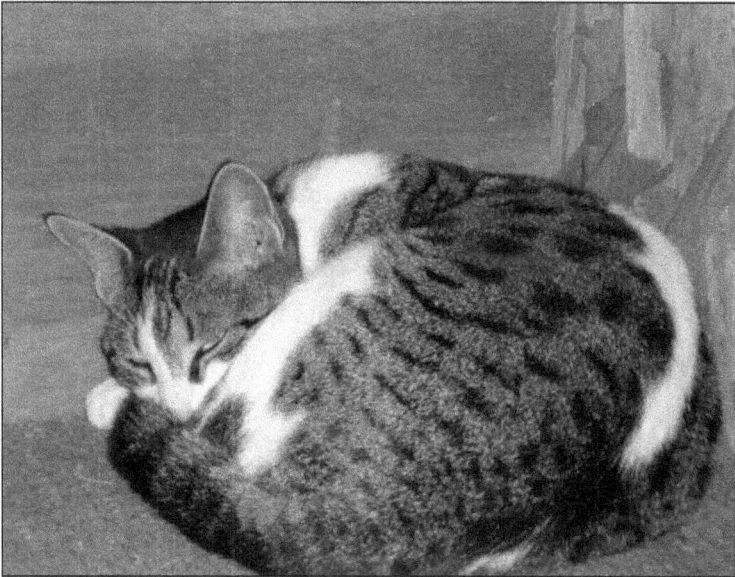

as they are unable to keep a dog. In modern life, cat is taking over the role of dog as man's best friend. Cats have adapted incredibly to a variety of environments and lifestyles, surviving and even thriving in extremes of temperature and harsh conditions. Whenever you keep the cat as a companion, keep in mind that it is likely to spend at least 14 years with you, possibly even more. You need to give careful thought while choosing the right type of kitten for you and your family.

Choosing the Right Type of Cat

Unlike dogs, most cats are the same size and shape, but there are differences, which are important to consider in choosing the right type of cat for you. Do not forget to keep in mind the needs of the cat, which include making sure the cat fits into the environment you will be able to provide. Following are some of the important points which should be kept in mind while choosing the cat:

(*a*) Time for Cat

Time is very important factor *i.e.*, it is important to consider how much time you can spend with your cat on day to day basis. Cats should be groomed regularly as cats with longer hair coats become more easily matted and require more frequent brushing and sometimes bathing, if necessary. Hairballs can be more of a problem too, if you do not groom your cat enough. Cats with short hair require regular bathing to remove the excess natural oils from the skin.

(*b*) Activities of Cat

Some breeds like Persians and Ragdolls are known for their laid-back attitude. These cats are content to sit and

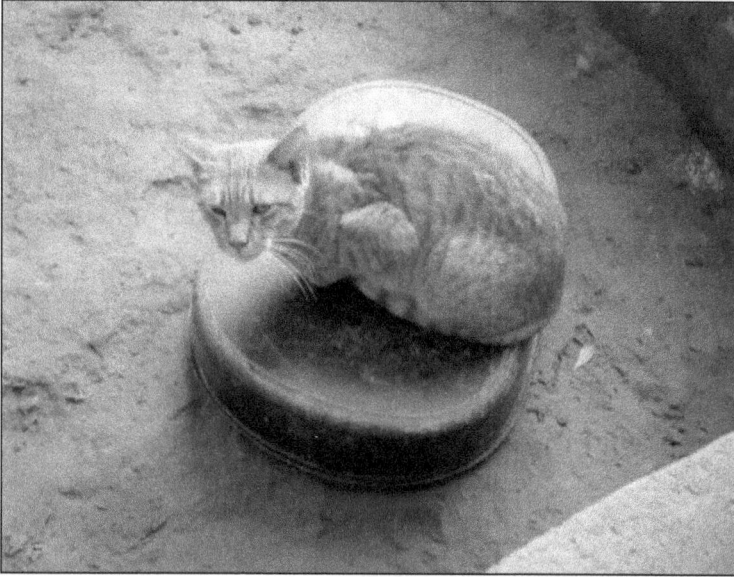

watch the world. If you want a cat to be with you while you sit, read a book or watch TV, these breeds are good choices for you. On the other hand, Siamese and Abyssinian breed cats are very active and will be with you wherever you are. It will take you longer to make the bed or to do other work as the cat tries to help you out.

(c) Children or Other Pets

Kittens who were exposed to children and other animals at 2 weeks of age will be best suited to live in a house with children and other pets. Some of the selective breeds have a tendency to do better with children and other pets.

(d) Sex of a Cat

Some prefer a female or a male cat. If you already have a cat, which is spayed or neutered, it is best to get a cat of the opposite sex. Different behavior problems are more common depending upon the sex of the cat. Unneutered male cats have behavioral problems of urine spraying. Unspayed female cats may vocalize and roll when they come into heat, which can frustrate many owners. It is suggestive to owner to get their pet cat spayed or neutered, which will prevent the other diseases also.

(*e*) Age of Cat

It is always a two ways decision to adopt a kitten or an adult cat. There are disadvantages in starting with a kitten or an adult cat. You may not be able to predict the future personality of a kitten. Cats are just like human beings as the traits of their personality are a result of their genetic background.

A kitten should be at least 9 weeks of age at the time of adoption and some even suggest 12 weeks of age before adoption. A kitten needs a longer period with its mother and other siblings to help it to learn normal and acceptable behavior.

A kitten that finds herself in a loving home where she can interact with people during play, grooming and other times will have different personality than other kitten which was kept as an outdoor cat and fed occasionally. So by choosing kittens you have chance to make effect on their personality than if you start with an adult. A kitten demands more time as they have to grow through different phases like climbing over the curtains, drapes and entering every open door or cupboard. They require more trips to the Vet for vaccinations, deworming and neutering as well. The selection of an adult cat bypass most of these phases. Taking care of a cat is a life time commitment. So you may choose a kitten or an adult cat according to your lifestyle.

(f) Purebreed or Crossbreed

It is totally your liking and choice whether you want a purebreed or crossbreed cat.

Purebreed Cats

If you want a cat with a specific appearance, you probably will look for selectively breed cat with that appearance in mind.

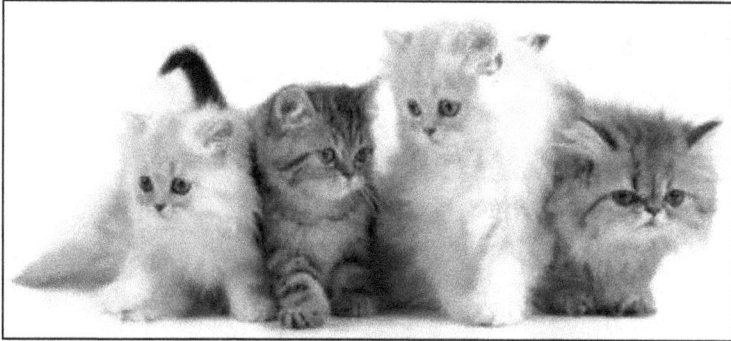

Crossbreed Cats

Crossbreed cats may have some disadvantages over the pure breed cats. These cats have man-made alterations in the basic structure. DO NOT forget the cost involved in buying a pure breed cat while domestic cats are available for free or with small adoption fee.

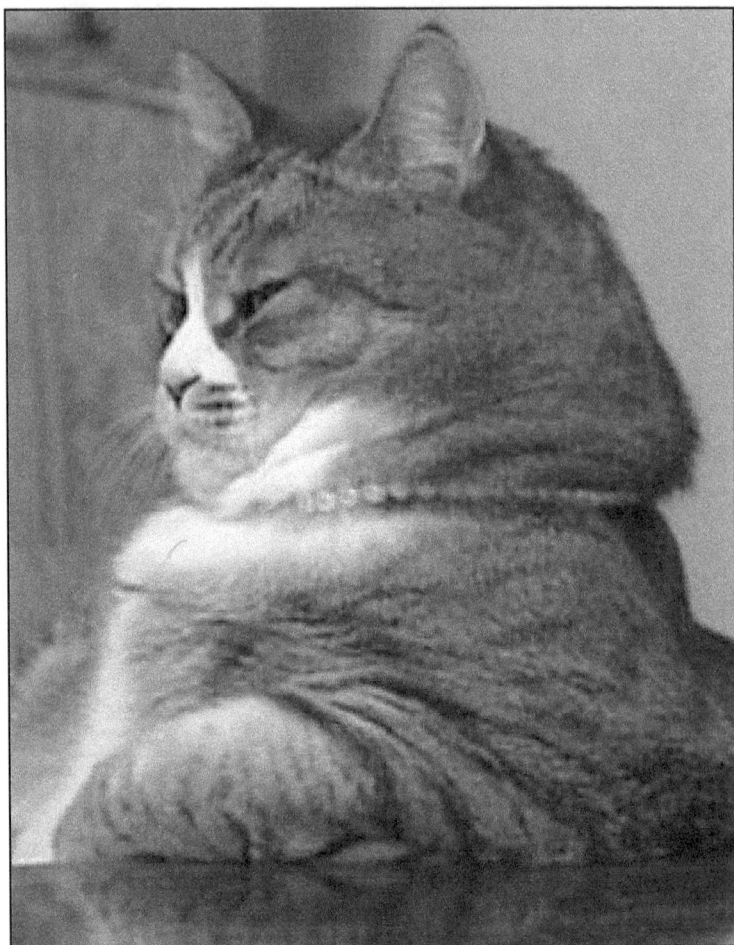

Chapter 2
Source to Look for a Cat

You can either buy or adopt a kitten or an adult cat from an animal shelter. Pedigree kittens may be available at pet stores or at home of some owners.

Animal shelter can be a good source for adoption of a kitten or an adult cat. Shelters may differ in the services they provide, which is often associated with their operating budgets. Despite budget, in shelters there are staffs who are dedicated to their work and the animals in their care.

Reasons for Animals in Shelters

Most of the pets are in shelters because the owners can no longer care for them for a variety of reasons:

☆ Owners may have health problem.

☆ They may be moving and cannot take the pet with them.

☆ Owner may become incapacitated or died.

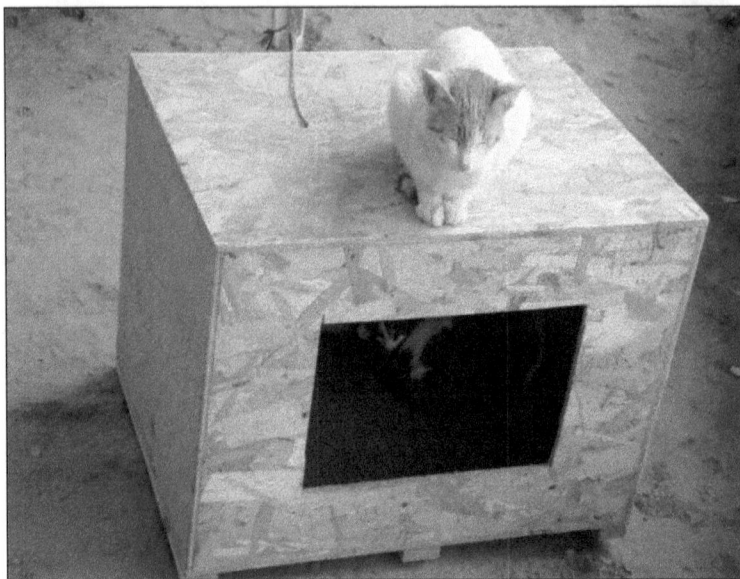

☆ They may have other pets who do not get along
   with this one.

☆ Owners do not have time for the pet due to change
   in lifestyle *e.g.* ill member, new baby, etc.

Before you Adopt a Cat

Adopting a pet cat is a big and life time commitment.
The cat will spend years of her life with you. So before you
go to a shelter and adopt a cat, you should ask yourself
following questions:

What type of pet I want e.g. breed, species or size,
gender, age, energy level? Be sure what characteristics you
want in your pet cat. So many people who come to shelter
with one type of pet in mind and fell in love with entirely
different type of pet and adopt him. Sometimes it work

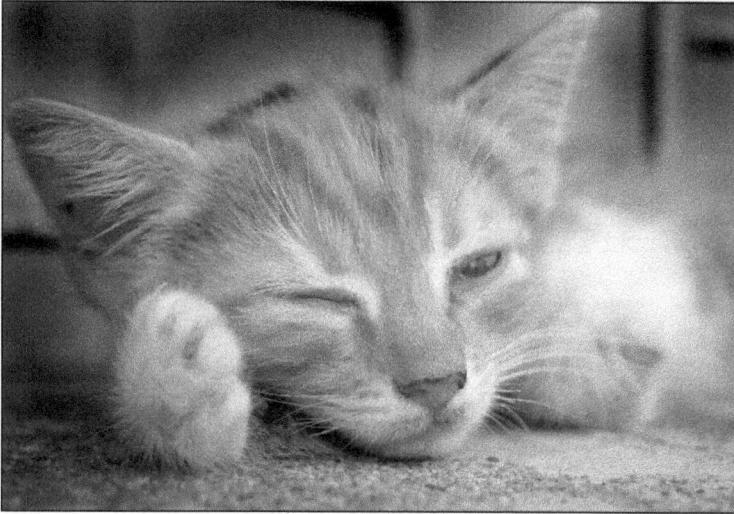

might out and other times it was just a moment decision. So be sure to decide what you are looking for.

Am I emotionally, personally and financially ready to take the responsibility of having a pet?

Do I understand the nutritional, health and housing requirements of the pet?

All of the family members agree about getting a new pet?

Choosing a Cat

When you go to a shelter for choosing a cat, you may be overwhelming to see the number of animals you can choose from. Always take your list of desired characteristics like size, sex, age, coat and temperament etc. to remind you of any limitations you have on your choice of animal. A caged cat may behave differently than a free cat in a home environment. So do not overlook the animals which

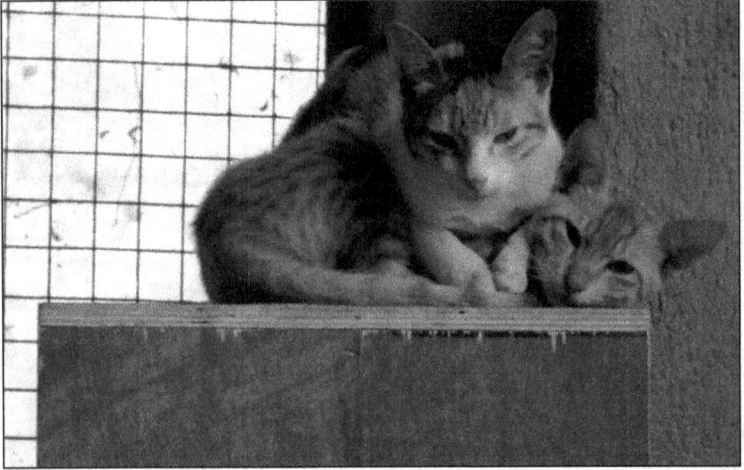

may appear quiet, scared or excited. You may ask the shelter staff regarding the animal's temperament and behavior and take the animal to a quiet place where you may be able to observe the cat's personality. It is imperative that the whole family should meet the pet, including children and other pets, so that the whole family can judge the temperament of animal.

Queries by an Animal Shelter

The animal shelter's staff may enquire following questions and it may include provisions that you:

- ☆ Will keep the cat as a domesticated pet.
- ☆ Provide good housing, health care and nutrition.
- ☆ Will get the pet neutered or spayed.
- ☆ Have permission from your landlord to have a pet
- ☆ Will not abandon the pet for any reason and will return the animal to shelter if you can not take care of cat.

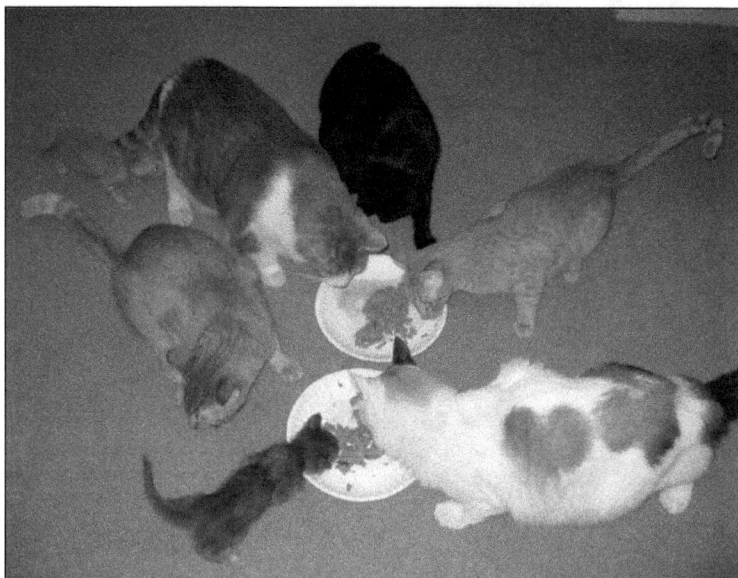

☆ Allow post adoption visits by the animal shelter.

☆ Do not have any history of animal abuse or negligence.

☆ Know that shelter will take the animal back, if mistreated.

☆ Have discussed the adoption issue with your family and they are agree on the new pet.

Pros and Cons of Adopting from Shelters

Pros

Shelters provide a wonderful mix of adoptable animals *i.e.,* purebreeds, mixbreeds, young or adult animals. You save your money as you don't have to pay to a breeder or pet shop. Another benefit is that people feel so happy that they could save the life of an animal by giving him a new and loving home. You can get good information on the

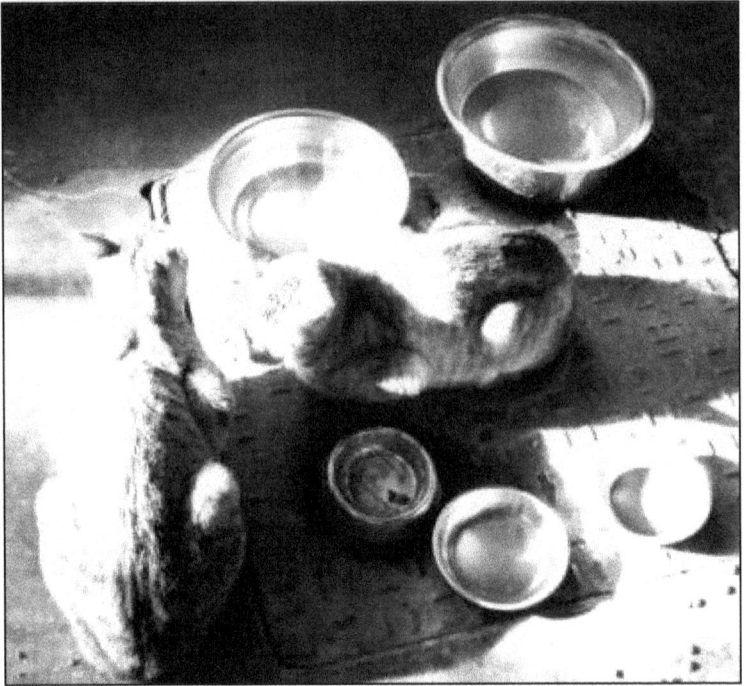

temperament and personality of the animal you want to adopt. You may even get his health records and an available description about his life in the former home. Some shelters neuter the animals before they put them for adoption. Most of the animals are dewormed, vaccinated, house trained and have basic training.

Cons

Animals in shelters are under stress. They may not be used to cages or other animals. They miss their old territory and their owners. Such animals may need extra care, love, patience, assurance and guidance. They may need your presence more than other animals that have come into your home. You may need to spend more time with her, play with her and to be with her when she explores new surroundings. Proving a crate to your new pet is a good idea as some pets find comfort in a small place.

Some animals may need special nutrition, depending upon their physical condition. Some animals may be too fat and others too thin. Some may have had very poor nutrition. Always ask the shelter what they fed your pet and continue with the same feeding at least for a week, as your pet adjusts at your home. If you need to or want to change the diet, do it slowly.

Though shelter staff will try to bathe and groom your pet before you receive him. But you may need to spend extra time for grooming your pet at first, as shelters may have limited time and facilities. So make this period as a happy and fun time and it will be a good time for you to make a bond with your pet.

Your pet needs a lot of adjustments to make, so train it slowly with lots of patience, affection and firmness. Regularity and consistency is also very important. Make sure that everyone uses the same command in the same manner.

Chapter 3

How to Choose Your Kitten: Personality and Health

You need to consider the personality of the kitten you want, its health and appearance.

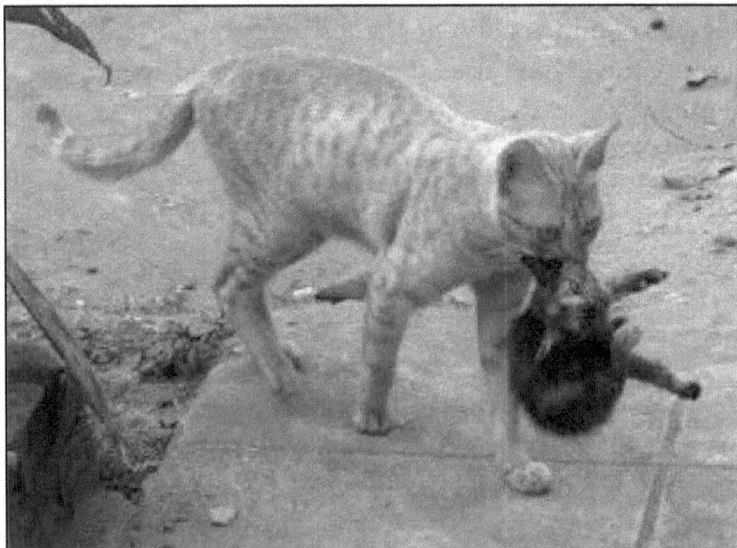

Mother and Kittens

It is best to choose a kitten from a litter, if get a chance. Observe the interaction between the kitten and mother as it may help you to choose a kitten with the traits you want. If the kittens sense fear of people in their mother, they may be fearful too. So adopting a kitten from a wild cat can be problematic for people who do not have an experience of handling cats.

Hand-reared or Orphan Cats

Kittens that do not grow up with the mother or other siblings are more likely to have behavior problems as they become adult. In a family, they learn how to cope with frustration; they learn guidelines as to what acceptable behaviour is and what is not. They come to know that biting and scratching is not tolerated. Hand-reared or orphan cats are more prone to displaying such unacceptable behaviors.

Early Socialization

Handling of the kitten from birth has great impact on the development of the kitten. Kitten who are handled

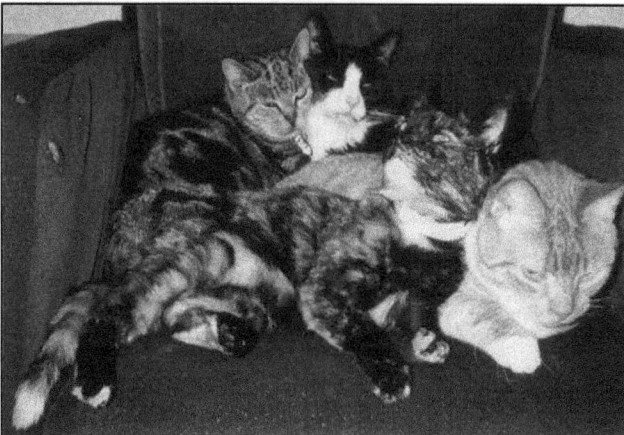

gently and multiple times a day and exposed to humans and animals at 2-9 weeks of age, are friendly and well adjusted and generally get along with humans and other animals. Kittens who did not have any human or animal contact during this period, or who are played with roughly or mistreated, may be more aggressive or timid.

So, if possible, find a litter that has been in a home environment, and used to the different smells, sights and sounds that are very common in a home. As such kitten will be less fearful of these noises than those who are not exposed until they are older.

Assessing Kitten Personality

A kitten should be playful but not too aggressive. In selecting a specific kitten, watch how the kittens interact with each other. Avoid kittens that hide in the corner or appear to bully their siblings.

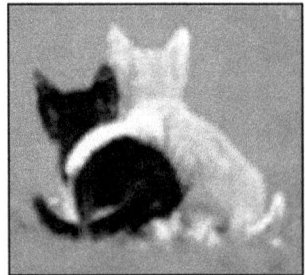

Kitten should be confident and not reluctant to come to you. Kittens that hiss or hide when approached by humans will be much more difficult to raise into friendly cats. Kittens should readily accept playing with you. It should not cower or show fear when petted on his head.

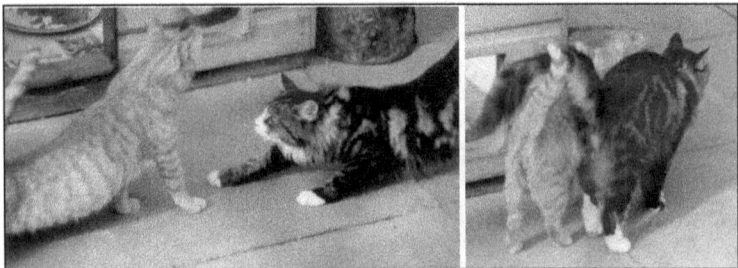

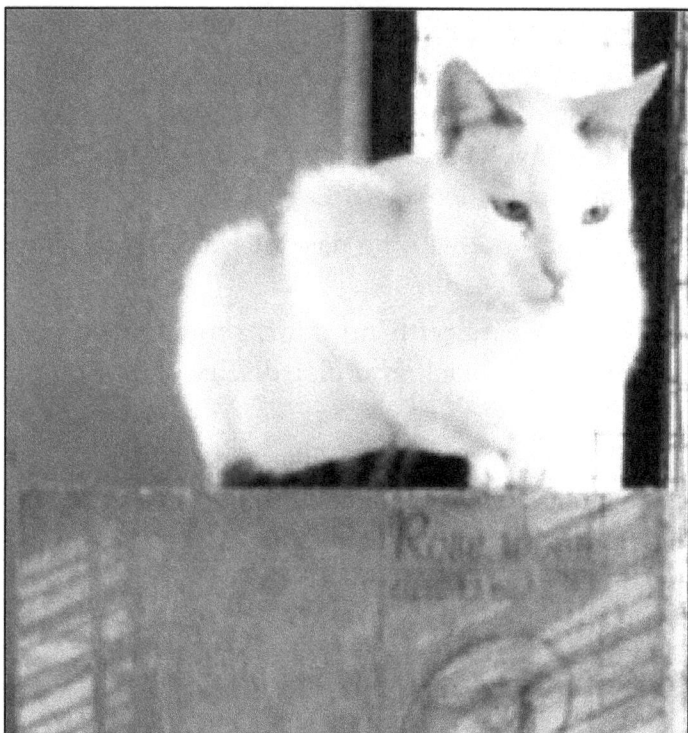

To find out the playful kitten, take a string along and drag it on the floor. Well-adjusted and healthy kittens should eagerly pounce on it and want to play. If the kittens have just had a rousing game of tag or wrestling, they may be tired. Kittens are often either very active or sleeping, not much in between.

Assessing Health

There are some obvious things to check for to be sure the kitten you select is healthy. However, always have your kitten checked by your Veterinarian, preferably the day you get the kitten.

A healthy kitten should have the following:

☆ Clear eyes with no tears or discharge. The eyes should be fully open, focus normally, and be able to follow your finger or a piece of string dragged across the floor.

☆ Clean nose with no nasal discharge, sneezing or labored breathing.

☆ Clean ears with no odor, scratching or head shaking. Black granular discharge indicate ear mites.

☆ The teeth should be white and properly aligned. Gums should be pink, with no sores or ulcers in the mouth or on the tongue.

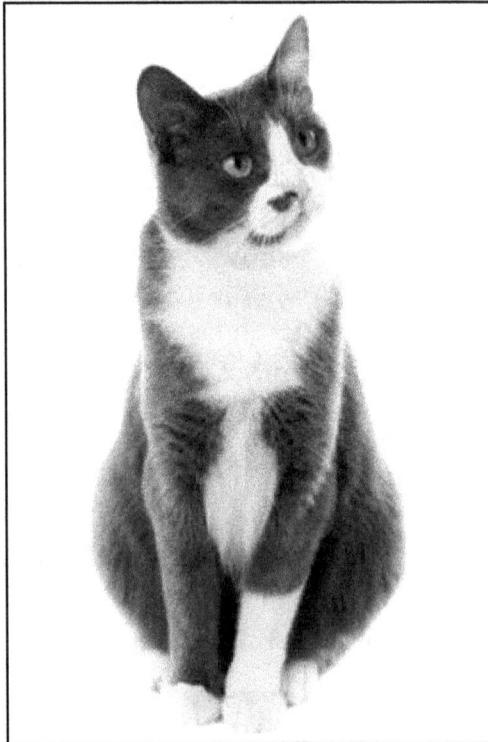

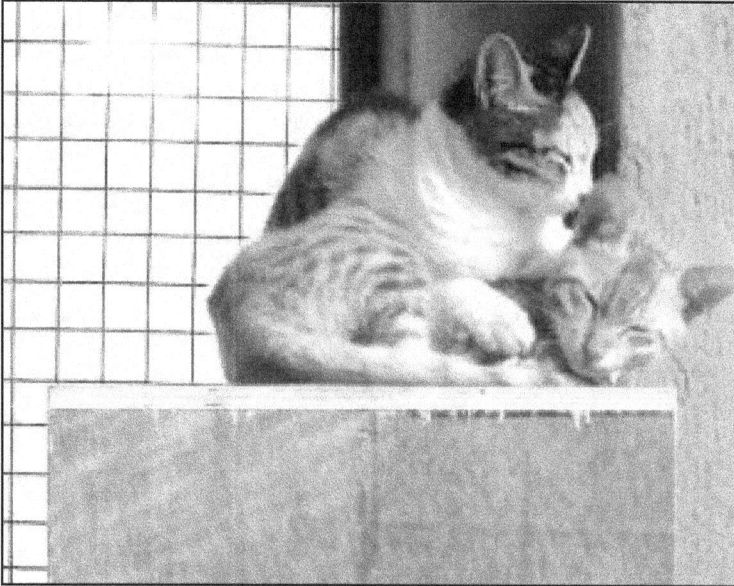

☆ Anal area should be clean, with no discoloration, matted fur or parasites.

☆ A clean, soft coat with no dandruff. There should be no evidence of external parasite, *i.e.*, lice or fleas, no evidence of scratching or bald spots. A kitten's coat will usually not appear as glossy as an adult's.

☆ A symmetrical body shape *i.e.*, neither too thin nor has a protruding belly.

☆ A good appetite and be fully weaned.

☆ No lumps or bumps, coordinated movements, with no head tremors. Some cats may have extra toes but usually it does not cause any problem.

Chapter 4

Kitten

Sexing of a Kitten

It can be difficult to tell the sexes apart when kittens are tiny. It is quite easier as they grow up. In a male kitten,

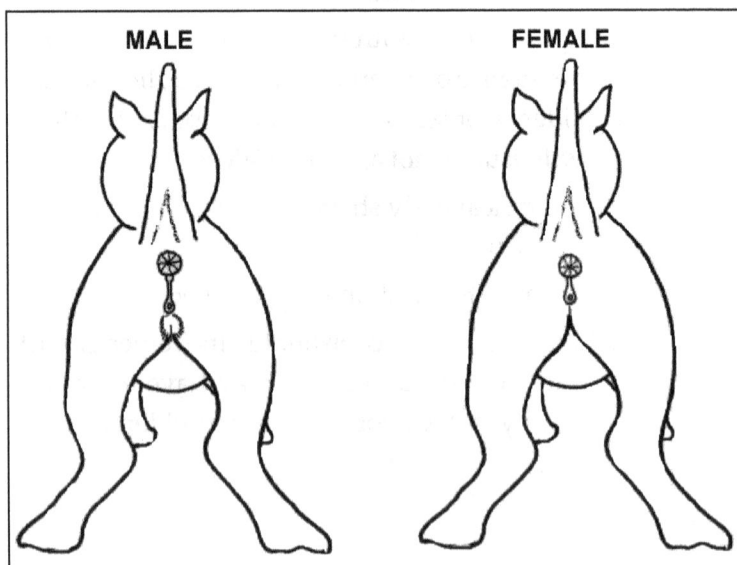

MALE   FEMALE

the tip of the penis is hidden in an opening 1 cm below the anus, with the scrotal sacs in between.

In a female kitten, the vulva is vertical slit almost joined to the anus like a letter "i".

Most of the differences between sexes are dominated by reproductive hormones. We can remove the influence of these hormones by getting them neutered before they become sexually mature *i.e.*, at or before six months of age. Once they are neutered, there is very little difference between the sexes and their behaviors are very similar. But choice of sex may be affected as if you will be introducing your kitten into a household where there is already a resident cat. So it is usually better to choose a kitten of the opposite sex to the older cat in order to remove any sexual competition.

If you plan to obtain two kittens together, it is best to choose one of each sex or two females to avoid the risk of competition, which can develop between males as they mature. Neutering will remove difference in behavior of males and females, but if done at proper age.

How Many Kittens?

The dog is a pack animal and need a group to live, whereas the cat is a solitary hunter. But pet cat's need to hunt can be removed by a ready supply of food at home. Cats normally sleep for up to 60 per cent of their lives and spend one-third of their waking hours grooming themselves, but still have time for interaction with other cats or with their human owners.

Most of the first time owners consider that adoption of a single kitten is enough, but there are advantages to obtain

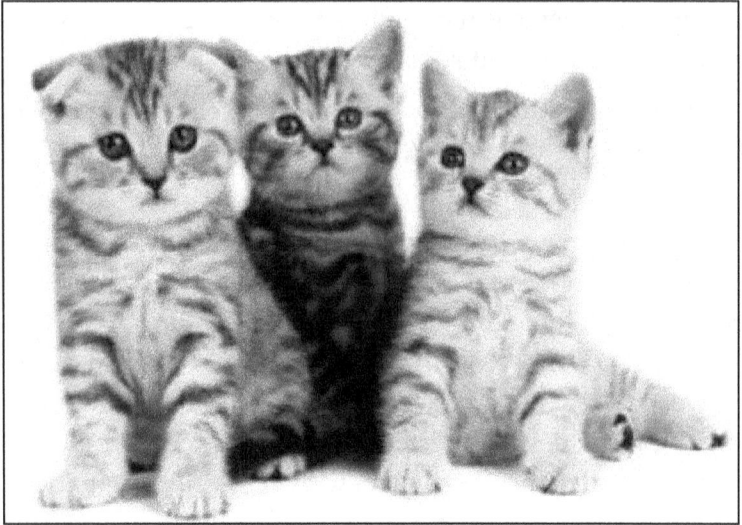

two kittens together. They usually think about the cost of feeding, neutering, vaccinations and medical expenses, but there are some non-cost related benefits *i.e.* the two kittens easily learn about the world around them.

Advantages

It is fun to have two kittens as you will see more of the feline behavior as they play. You get a wonderful opportunity to see how much they can confront themselves or erect their fur on various body parts during play-fights. The personality of every kitten is individual; if one kitten is a little nervous and quiet, another may be less-inhibited. Obtaining two kittens together removes many of the problems of introducing a companion at a later date. Once one cat has acquired territorial attachments, it is much harder to get two cats to share together and adjust. Companionship will be of particular help in those first few days on entering a new home, when all is strange and very frightening. Getting two kittens together – sometimes it is the trouble, but the fun factor is also associated.

Disadvantages

Some people want dog-like devotion from their cats. Cats do not spurn our attention because they have been curled up with their feline partners all day, but will seek out a warm lap whenever it becomes available. Another disadvantage may be extra time and effort required to groom long-haired kittens.

Routine Veterinary Examination for Kitten

There are few important things to keep your kitten happy and healthy. It is advisable to take your kitten to Veterinarian for regular checkups. The first visit should be on the day when you are bringing your new kitten home.

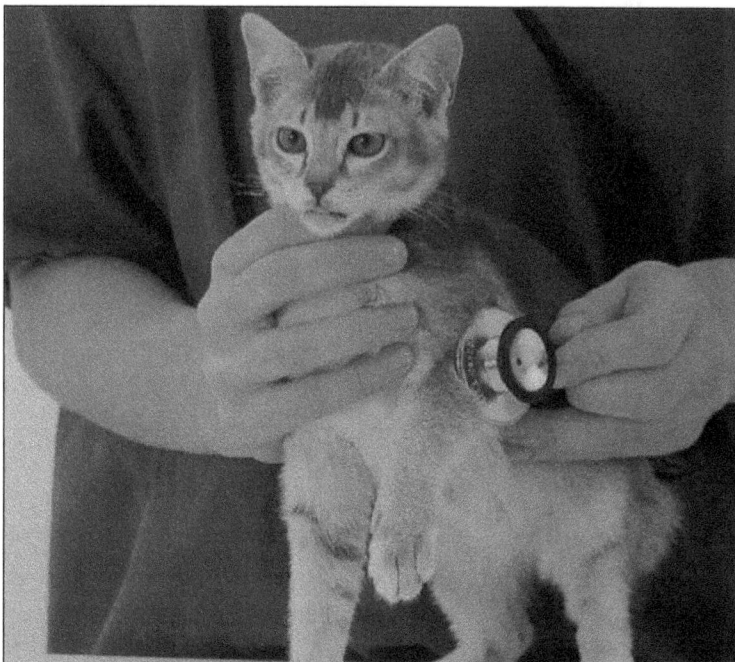

A visit to your Veterinarian usually covers a lot more than vaccinations. Always make a list of specific questions you have prior to the exam.

First Visit

☆ General examination of your kitten.

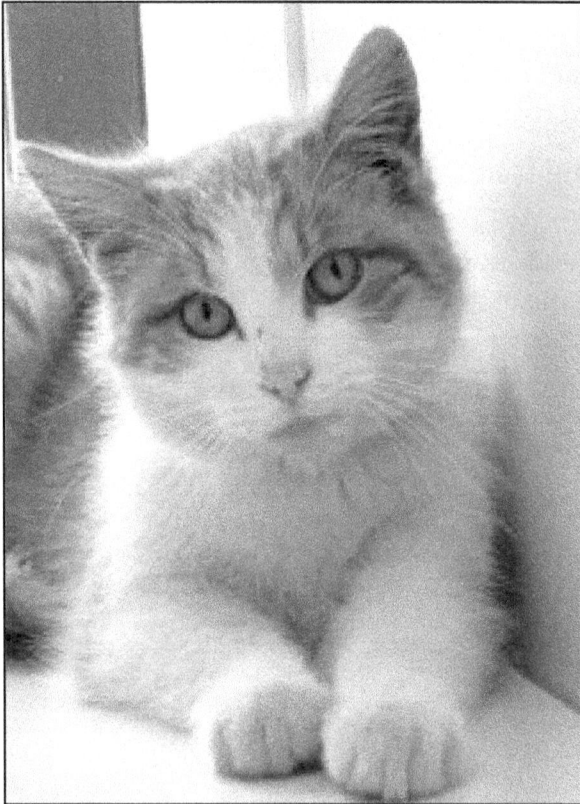

☆ Weighing your kitten.

☆ Deworming of your kitten. Inform the Veterinarian about previous deworming and if your kitten was exposed to other cats.

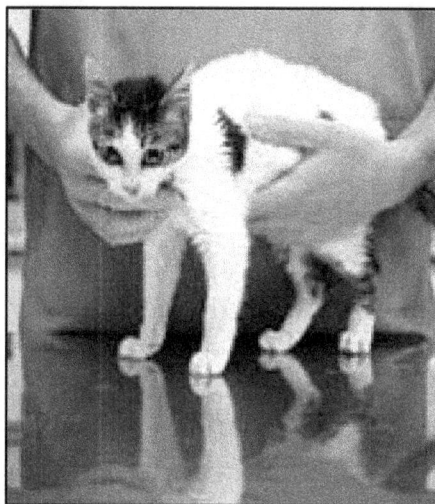

☆ Get your kitten checked for parasites – both external and internal.

☆ Discuss vaccinations and have the proper ones given.

☆ Discuss feeding your kitten – how much, how often, dry or canned.

☆ Discuss grooming and care of skin, coat, eyes, ears and nails.

☆ Discuss about dental hygiene and daily care.

☆ Discuss flea and tick control medications and start if necessary.

☆ Discuss normal kitten behavior, any problem behaviors and litter box training.

☆ Discuss introduction of your kitten to other pets in your family and to children.

Second Visit

☆ General physical examination including weighing of your kitten.

☆ Have your kitten checked for external and internal parasites.

☆ Discuss any health issue and have your kitten dewormed.

☆ Discuss vaccinations and have the proper ones given.

☆ Discuss any changes or problems in feeding your kitten.

☆ Discuss grooming, oral hygiene or any other health concern.

☆ Review normal behavior or any change in behavior.

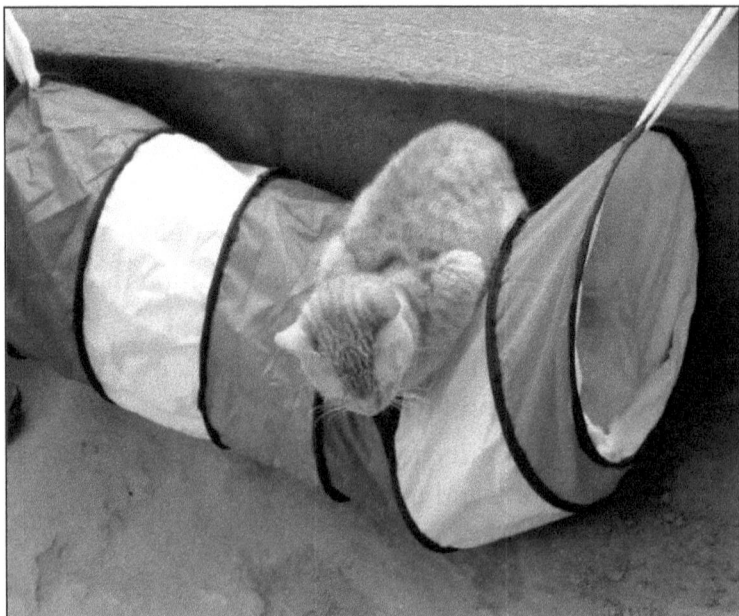

Subsequent Visits

☆ General physical examination including weighing of your kitten.

☆ Have your kitten dewormed and vaccinated.

☆ Discuss any health concerns and spaying or neutering your kitten.

☆ Discuss any problems in feeding your kitten.

☆ Discuss oral hygiene, grooming or other concerns.

☆ Discuss boarding facilities, traveling with your kitten or other concerns.

As your kitten grows into an adult, it should have an annual exam. As these exam are not only for vaccinations but also to evaluate the overall health of your pet.

Chapter 5
Kitten Supplies

Before getting a new kitten, you will need:

☆ Cat carrier

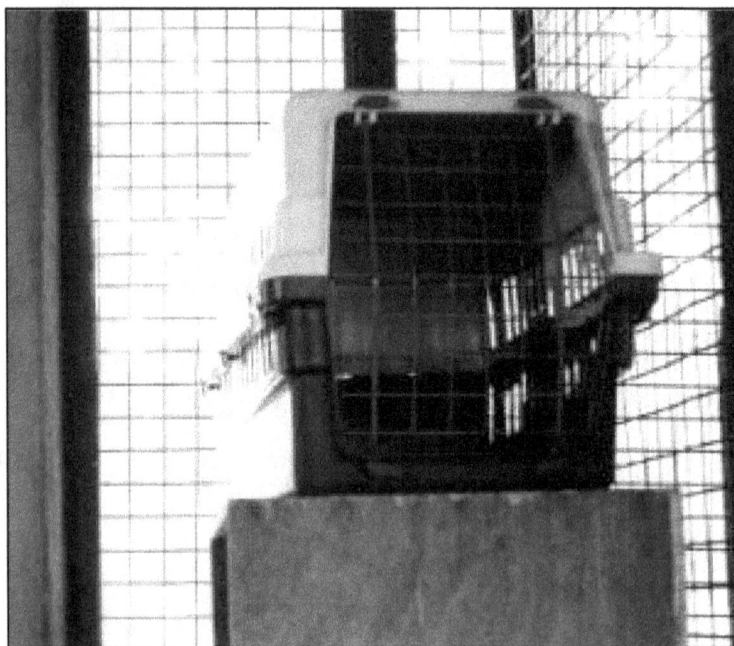

☆ Cat bed

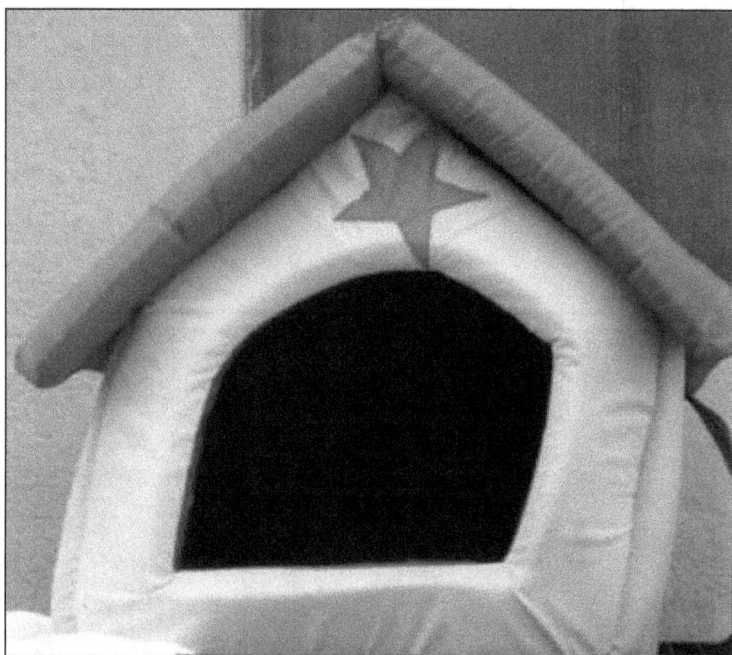

☆ Food and water bowls

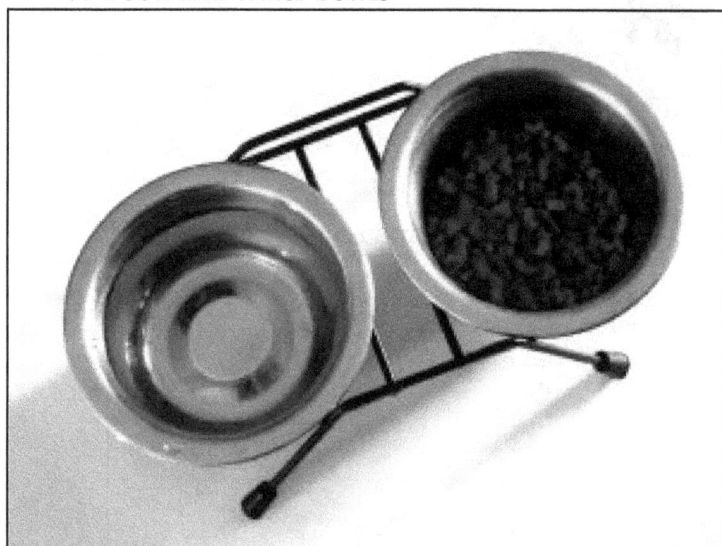

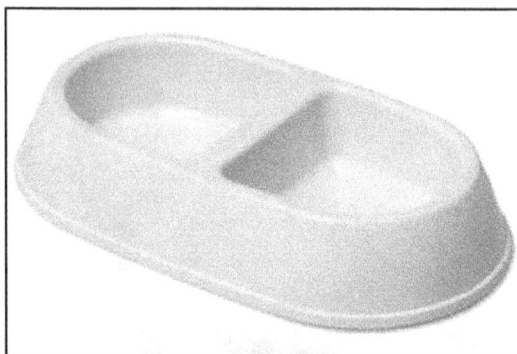

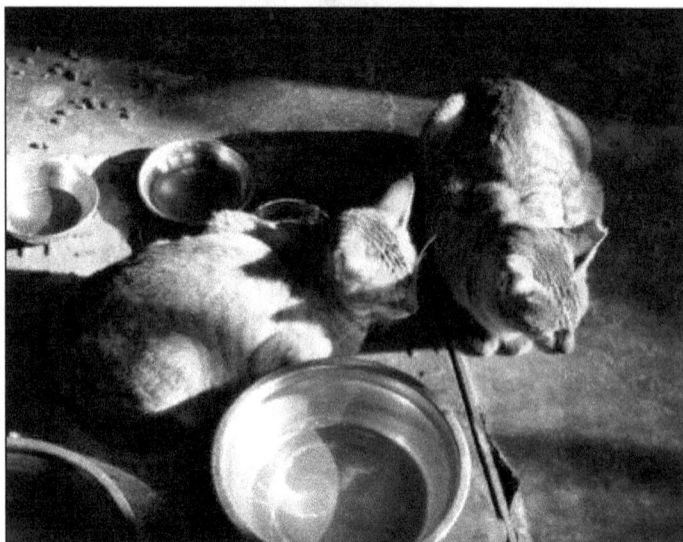

☆ Food-dry or canned

☆ Litter box, litter and scoop

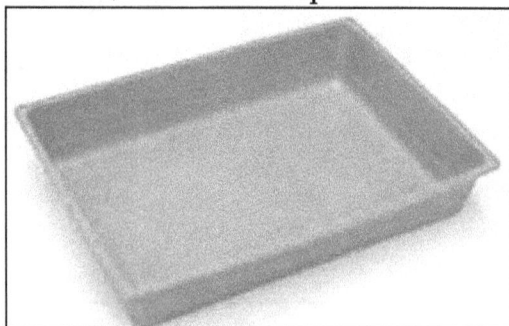

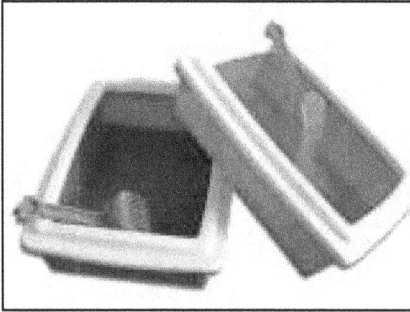

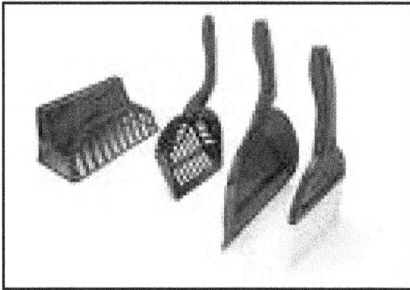

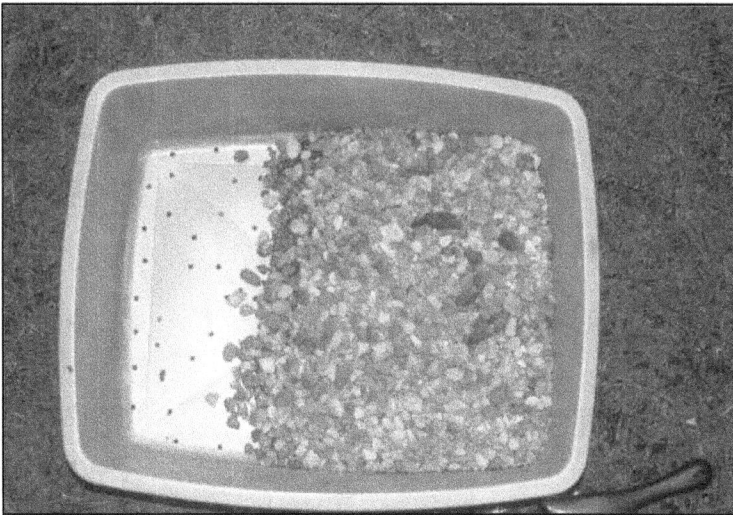

☆ A collar and a tag

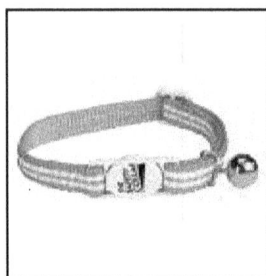

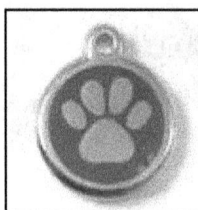

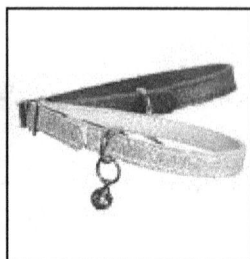

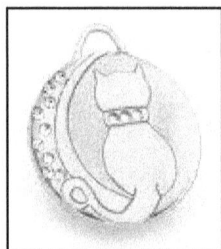

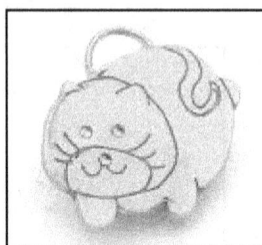

☆ A scratch post and toys

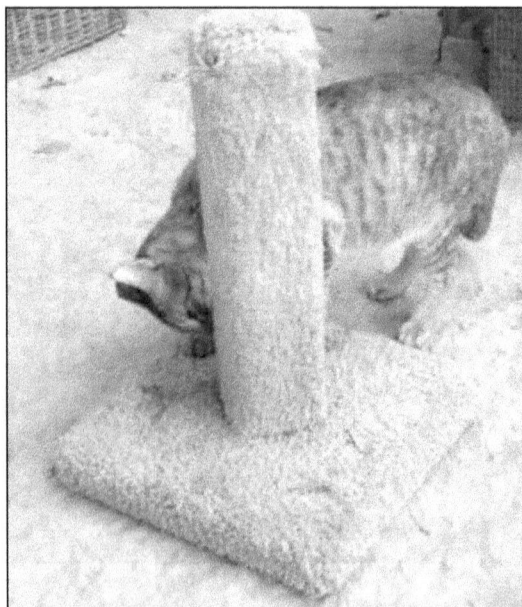

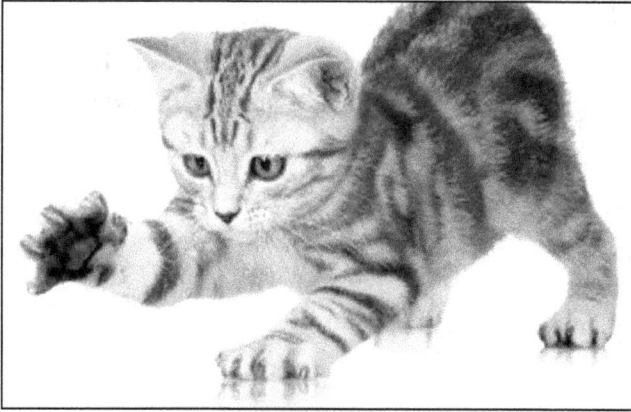

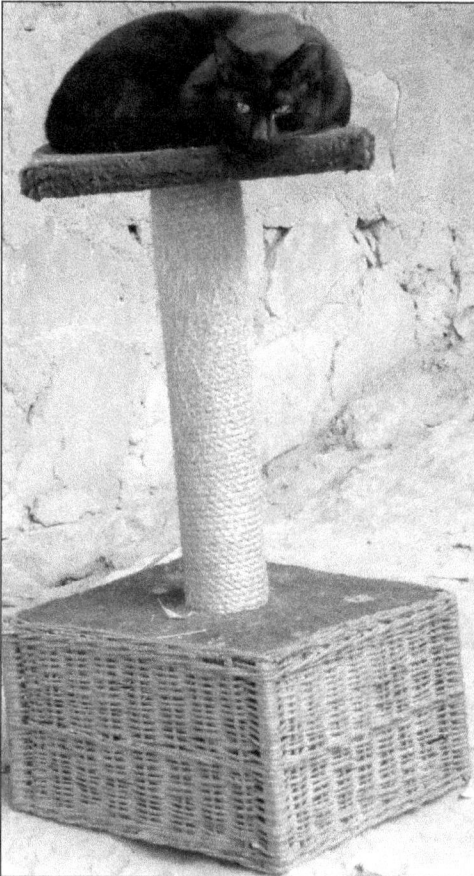

☆ Grooming supplies, according to the breed of cat.

☆ Health care supplies, which will include ear cleaner, cat toothbrush and toothpaste.

Chapter 6
Bringing Home a New Cat or Kitten

You might be feeling excited to bring home a new cat or kitten. You cannot wait to introduce the new companion to your family and friends and you are already looking forward to years of happy companionship. The way you introduce your new kitten or cat to your household can make a big difference in how well he/she makes the

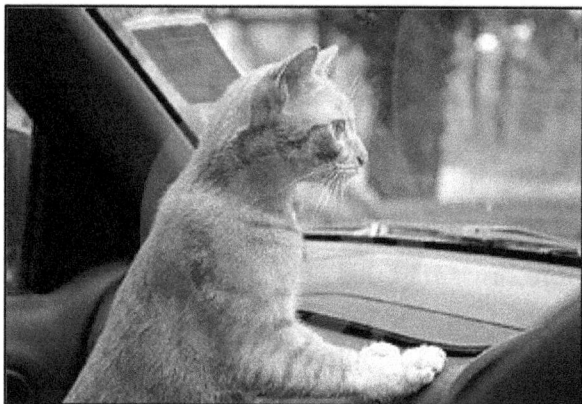

adjustment. Cats are habitual in nature and they like things to be predictable and almost the same from day to day. At your home with busy schedule the easiest going cat may feel stressed and nervous. To make it comfortable, take things slowly and give your cat plenty of time to get used to new home.

Before Bringing Your Cat or Kitten Home

You should prepare some plans and changes at your home to make it easier for you and your cat. First, make an appointment with your Veterinarian for a complete examination of your pet. Schedule it in such a fashion that you can take your cat to the Veterinarian immediately after picking him up.

Make sure to have a sturdy travel crate for the cat to ride in. Cats may feel nervous in the car; they may feel more secure in an enclosed space. An unrestricted cat may climb down by the pedals or jumps on to your shoulder. Try to keep your cat in a carrier; it will be helpful if the cat vomits, urinates or defecates, which some cats will do if they are nervous.

Make arrangements, if possible, by bringing a towel for the cat to sleep on for several days before you pick her up. The sense of smell is very important to cats and it will make them more comfortable to have something that smells like their former home. Place the towel in the carrier for the ride home and leave it in the carrier for your new pet to sleep on the first few days.

Before bringing your new pet cat home, put his food, water, toys, scratching post and litter pan in a room you can close. To limit the number of changes for your pet, find out what food and litter the cat has had and try to get the same.

The Initial Introduction to Home

Cat need to become familiar and comfortable at new home. For a new cat whole house can be overwhelming and it may hide under beds or furniture for days. It will be much less stressful for your cat to learn about you, your family and your home at a time. It is even more important if there are multiple people or pets in your household.

When you bring your cat home, place it in the room you have fixed up for him, keep this room closed off and let him explore that area first. Let the cat come out of his crate on his own, do not try to force him out. Usually cats are curious and will soon come out to explore their surroundings. If the cat seems very timid, you can leave the room for a while and can come back later. Whenever the cat is ready to come out, stay where you are and let him come to you. Talk in a soft tone, pet him if it seems interested, but do not try to pick him up. Give him time to learn that he can trust you.

Introducing to Other Family Members

Introduce other family members slowly. They should come into the room one at a time and play with the cat. Explain and show to younger children how to gently stroke the cat's fur and offer her a few treats. Make sure to tell them that they are not to chase the cat while he/she eats, sleeps or uses the litter box. If there are no other pets, you can let the cat begin to explore the rest of the house.

Introduction to Other Pets in Your Home

Before bringing a new cat in the house, take it to your Veterinarian for an exam as new cat may carry disease or parasites to other cats or dogs.

Pet Cats

Keep the new cat in a quiet, separate room if there are other cats in the house as they will quickly become aware of new cat's presence. The cats usually sniff at each other under the closed door. Do not be surprised of hissing. Try to feed them on either side of the door so that they will start associating the smell of the other cat with food. After some days take the new cat out of its room, put the old cat in that room with the door closed and let the new cat explore the rest of the house for a few hours each evening.

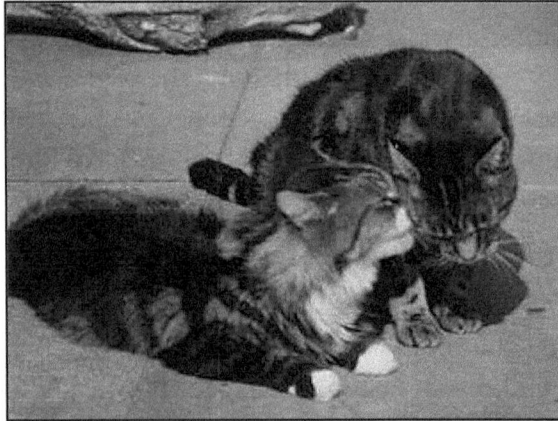

Now let the cats see each other, yet still keep them separated. After a few days of this, try feeding the cats together but at opposite ends of the room. Each day move the food dishes very slightly closer to each other. Until the cats are eating side by side. The main purpose behind this

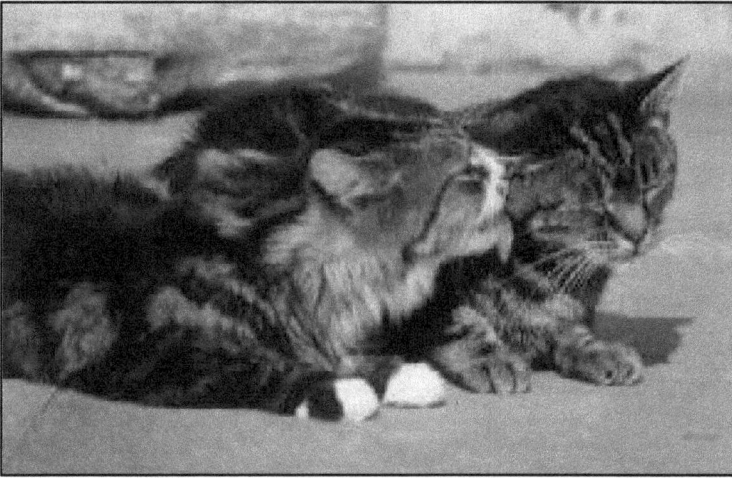

for the cats to associate each other with the pleasant experience of eating. When the cats are comfortable with each other open the door all the way, allowing the cats to come and go as they please. Try not to leave both cats alone until you are sure they will get along well. Always make sure to provide one litter box per cat. It will help to prevent a dominant cat from stalking the other and keeping him from using the litter box.

Pet Dog

Introduction of a new cat into a house with a dog is little different. Initially for the first few days keep them separated in different rooms. Then slowly leave the cat freely in the house whenever the dog is outside. When you feel that the cat is comfortable in the house, you can begin introducing the dog and the cat. Try to keep the dog on a short leash and give him the command for a sit or stay and then allow the cat to come inside the room. If the dog is quiet and the cat seems interested, let the cat come to the dog. Just be careful that the dog should not become aggressive or cat might claw at the dog's face. Monitor both the dog and cat closely and do not leave them unattended until you are sure that they will get along well. Make sure to keep litter boxes out of the dog's reach and also to prevent from eating feces.

Always take time to gradually introduce the new comer as it will increase the chances of your new cat becoming a happy and permanent member of your family.

Chapter 7
Selecting a Name for your Kitten/Cat

Selection of a name for your new kitten or cat is an important decision. The name will be used to relate to the cat for the rest of its life. Always select a proper name and keep the following suggestions in mind:

(a) *No names like commands*: Do not choose a name that sounds like a command. Pets rely on 'sounds like' rather than 'means' when they try to understand what we are communicating to them. Names like 'Rum', 'Joe' can end up sounding like 'come' or 'no'. Your cat may get confused which way to turn when you call.

(b) *Avoid same names*: Always try to avoid similar names for your family member and your cat. This would result in confusion for your cat.

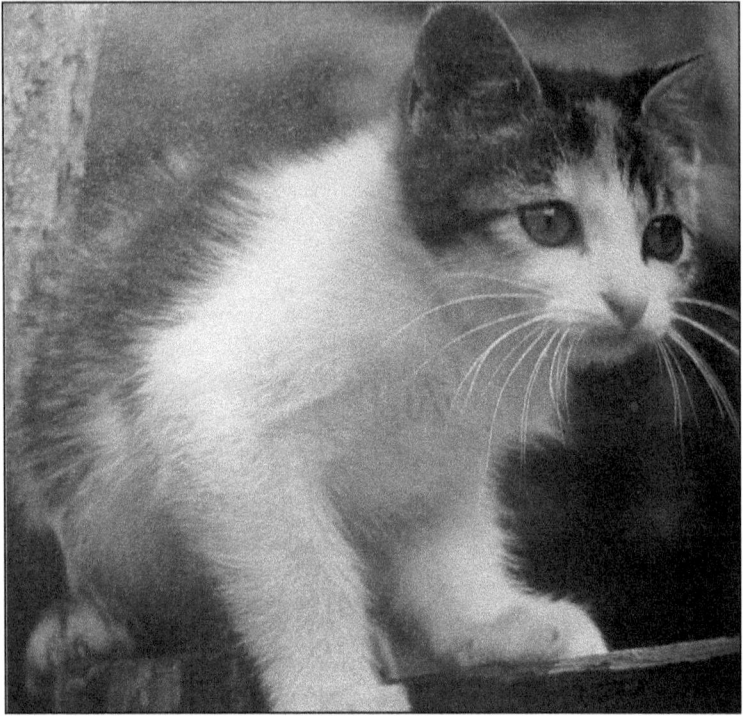

(*c*) *Short names*: Try to keep the short names as they will be easier for your cat to recognize than longer names.

(*d*) *Try to use hard consonants*: Hard consonants like k, d, and t are easier to hear and differentiate than soft consonants such as f, s or m. Thus names like Katy, Doucheka and Tibul are recognized easily than Shana, Merl or Fury.

(*e*) *Be comfortable to call the name in public*: Be sure to pick up the name you will feel comfortable calling in public. Try not to choose any funny name.

Chapter 8
Litter Box Training

As everything is ready at your home and you want to make your new cat comfortable at home. So along with providing food, a safe environment and love, it is important to give attention to cat's litter box. Elimination disorders are one of the biggest reasons for cats to be given up to shelters and one of the most common problem for which people seek Veterinary advice. Most cats will instinctively

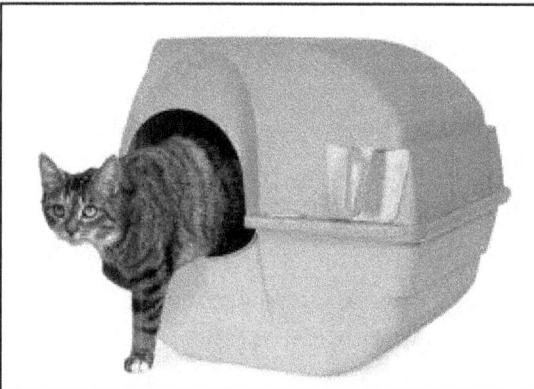

use a litter box from the time they are young kitten. Few basic tips about cat and litter boxes can help prevent problems from starting in the first place. Here are some important tips to keep in mind:

New Kittens

Kittens usually learn from observing their mothers and cats have a natural instinct to eliminate in sand or soil. Kittens usually start learning to use the litter box at 3 or 4 weeks of age. So you will not need to train the kitten as you would housebreak a puppy. It is important to make sure that your kitten knows the location of the litter box and it should not be placed in a noisy or hard-to-reach place.

After brining your kitten home, take it to the litter box at a quiet time. Place her into the litter box; gently take her front paws to show her how to scratch at the litter once or twice. If cat jumps out of the box, place her in the box when a cat would normally go to the bathroom: firstly in the morning, after meals, playing and waking up from a nap. Cats prefer privacy when using the litter box, so leave her alone while he/she is using the box. Most cats will make the adjustment to a new litter box without any problems. If there are any accidents, don't scold or punish your cat. Clean up the accident with an enzyme cleaner to remove stains and odor. After that, place the kitten in the litter box frequently until she starts using it. If you notice any diarrhea or straining, have your kitten examined by your Veterinarian to rule out any medical problems.

As per the thumb rule, you should provide one litter box per cat, plus one extra. Sometimes cats are fussy and they will not use a litter box that other cats have used. Some cats may prefer to use one box to urinate and other to defecate in.

Type and Size of Litter Box

In the market many types of litter boxes are available like covered boxes, self-cleaning boxes and boxes designed to fit into corners. Always keep in mind that kittens or old cats may need boxes with lower sides. You can also cut down the sides of the sweater box if needed. Some cats may feel secure in a litter box with a hood, but these boxes can concentrate odor and should be cleaned daily.

The automatic self-cleaning litter boxes can save on clean-up time. If you have several cats, you need to provide several types of litter boxes so that your cats can choose between them.

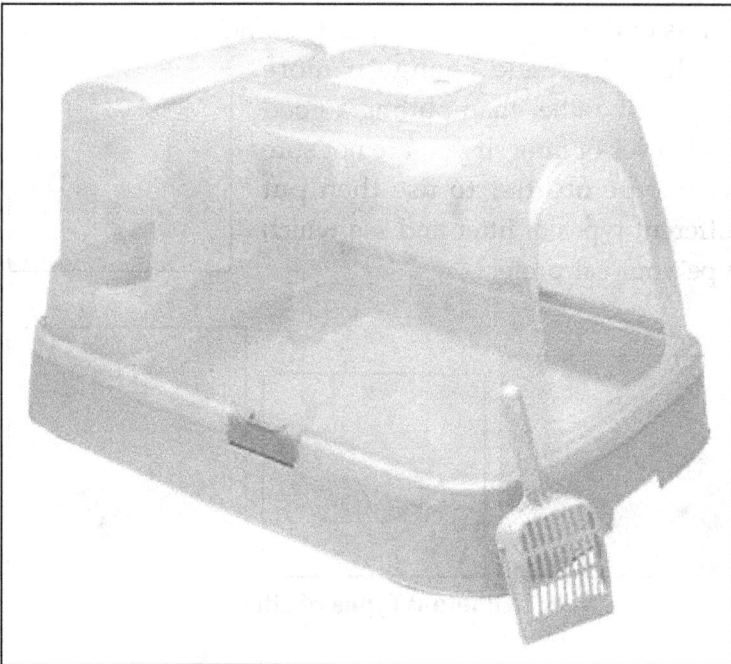

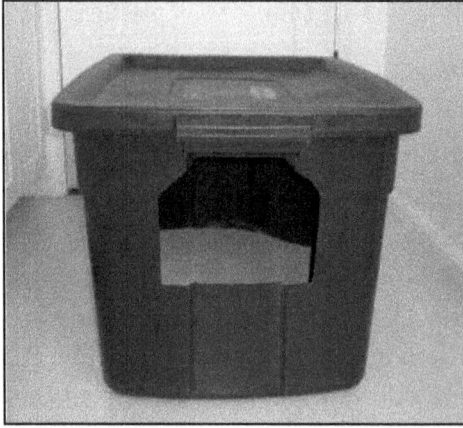

Litter

Cats prefer to use a litter that has the consistency of sand or soil and unscented litter than scented one. Two inches of litter in the box is usually sufficient. It is better to use less litter and change it more frequently rather than putting a good thick layer of litter. If you are not sure what type of litter to use then put different types of litter and see which type your cat prefer?

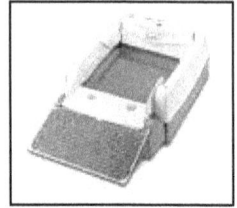

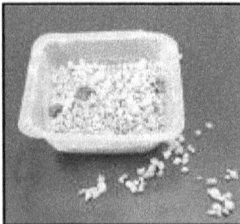

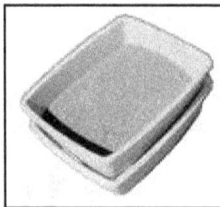

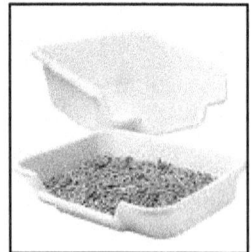

Different Types of Litter

Location

Cats usually prefer to use the litter box in a quiet, private place. Busy places, noises or people walking in that area or if disturbed by a dog or another cat, your cat may leave the litter box and may prefer to choose another location. If you have more than one cat, try to put the litter box in a location where one cat cannot corner another cat as she leaves the litter box. There should always be an entrance or an escape route.

Most of the cats do not prefer to have the litter box right next to their food dish, so avoid this type situation if possible.

Cleanliness

Though cats are extremely clean creatures and they may not use a litter box that is cleaned often and properly. Scoop the litter boxes at least once daily. Wash the litter box and change the litter completely once a week. Rinse the box well after washing it and do not clean the box with any smelling disinfectant. Regular cleaners may mask the odor so that we can't smell it, but to a cat the odor will be discernible and cat may continue to use that area as bathroom.

Chapter 9

Kitten Proofing your Home

Kittens are like babies which have a tremendous amount of energy and are very curious in nature. They love to play with new objects and may climb into small spaces or over the shelves. Their instinctive behavior could be very dangerous as they run and pounce on everything. So you should prepare your home for the following things:

☆ Keep all medications and toxic chemicals in cabinets away from kitten's reach.

☆ All toxic plants should be kept outside the home *e.g.* liliy, tulip.

☆ Lids in the toilets should be kept closed and never leave a filled bathtub or sink unattended.

☆ Use only safe cat toys and keep small objects out of your cat's reach.

☆ Always keep window screen securely fastened. Either tie up the excess cords or cut the loop in the cord.

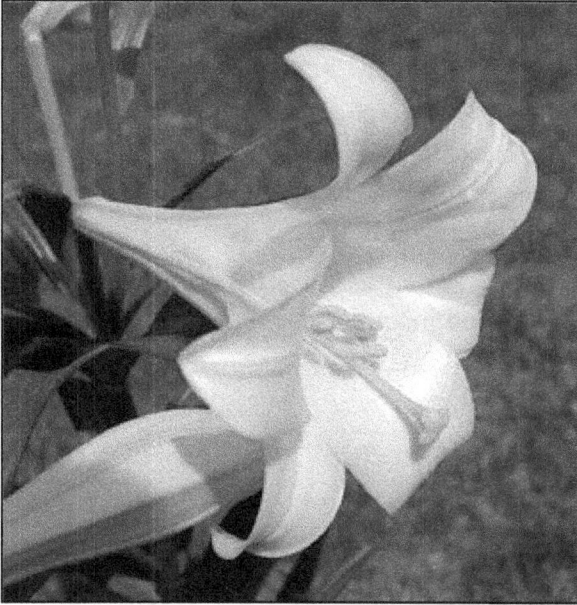

Lily

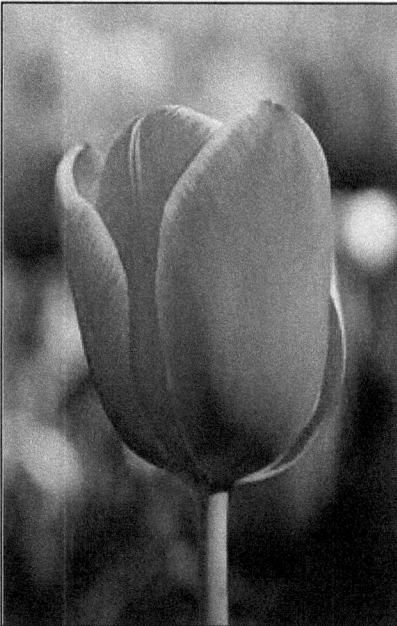

Tulip

☆ Keep the refrigerator door closed.

☆ Be careful in the kitchen about ovens as they can cause burns.

☆ Many human foods and fruits like grapes and tobacco products can be toxic to cats. So keep them out of your kittens' reach.

☆ Uncooked meat, poultry or fish can lead to infection in cats.

☆ Electric cords should not be kept loose as they can cause burns.

Chapter 10
Car Sickness

For some cats, car rides are a great deal of anxiety. A combination of fear and not knowing what is happening will cause drooling, shaking and vomiting in some cats. In humans we call it as car sickness or motion sickness. But true motion sickness is a result of an inner ear problem. However, the sickness is strictly an over-reaction to the fear and apprehension of the car noise, motion etc. So you can follow the below described steps to make your cat used to the car ride:

(a) Get Your Cat Used to the Car Environment

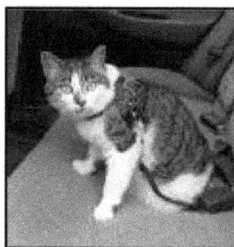

Take the cat in the car and give him a treat. Do not move the car; just spend some time with your cat in the standing car. Repeat this several times. If your cat is afraid of getting into the car, try feeding a treat close to the car.

(b) Get Your Cat Used to in Running Car

Repeat first step and then start the car. Give a treat before and after. If she is nervous, talk to his/her in an 'upbeat' fashion. Take your time and make sure he/she is relaxed before ending the seassion.

(c) Get Your Cat Used to Motion of Moving Car

After second step, back the car to the end of the driveway, then forward again to the garage. Give her a treat and praise her.

(d) Take His/Her to a Short Trip Around the Block

Treat and praise before and after, and calm, reassuring talk throughout the ride. Gradually increase the distance traveled until your cat is calm.

In severe cases, you may need to give them anti-anxiety drugs to make them calm. Get kittens used to the car while they are young and are more receptive to new adventures.

Chapter 11
Administering Medicines

Veterinarian may ask you to give medicines to your cat. Following guidelines will help you how to do it.

Administration of a Pill

The easiest way to give a pill is to hide it in a piece of food. You can use a small amount of butter, cheese, tuna, liver, canned food or semi-moist food. It is best to give a small amount of the food without the pill first. It is advisable not to mix the medication in an entire meal as if the cat does not eat the whole meal, she will not get the appropriate dose of medication.

If your cat is not taking the pill in food, then you should follow the following steps:

1. Get the pill out of the bottle and bring the cat to the place where you want to give the medicine
2. Ask helper to hold the cat. If you are right handed person, then put left hand over the head of cat

and press mouth with thumb and first finger to open it.

3. Now place one of free fingers of the hand holding the pill between the lower canine teeth and push down.

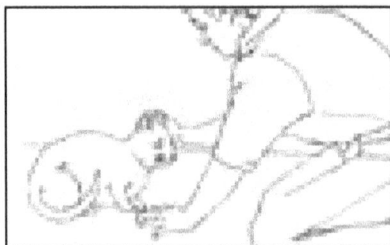

4. Now quickly place the pill as far back in your cat's mouth as possible, getting it over the hump of the tongue. Do not place your hand too far in or your cat may gag.

5. Close cat's mouth, hold it closed and lower his/ her head to a normal position, which will make

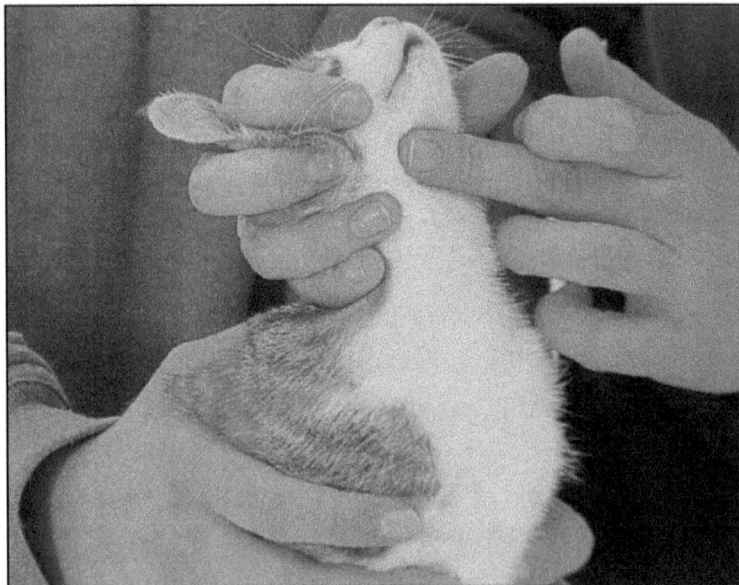

swallowing easier. Gently rub or blow on cat's nose as it will stimulate a cat to lick her nose, and then swallow.

6. Talk with your cat or give his/her some treat to make it easier for next time. The quicker you give the medicine, the easier it is for both of you.

If you still have problems, then ask your Veterinarian or staff to demonstrate it.

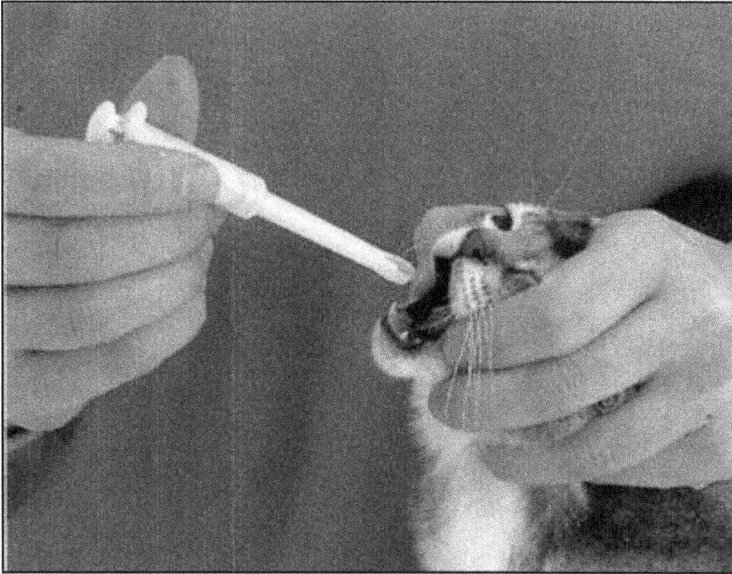

Administering Liquid Medicine

Medication can be given with food. If the dose is small, mix it with a small amount of canned food. It is best not to mix the medicine in entire meal, as he/she may not eat the whole meal and then he/she will not get the full dose of medication.

You can adopt the following steps for administration of medicine:

1. Shake the bottle before use if necessary and get the medication ready in the dropper or syringe.

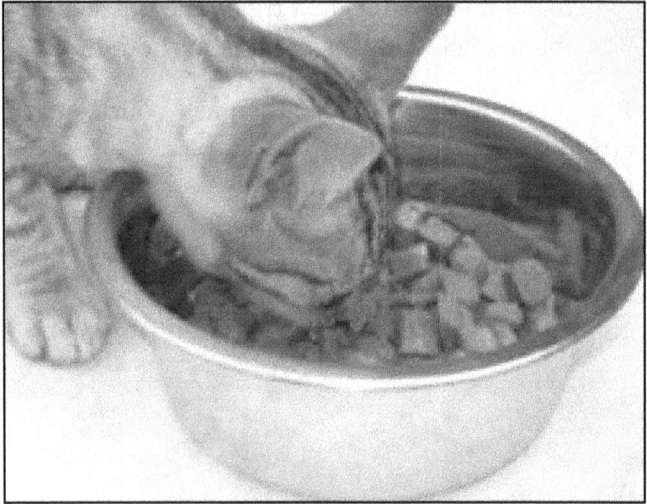

2. Bring your cat to the place you want to give the medication. It is helpful to wrap the cat in a towel or blanket so that just her head is sticking out. Try to place her back end against something so that she can not back away from you.

3. Now pick up the syringe or dropper in your working hand and with your other hand, gently grasp your cat's head from above with your thumb on one side of the hinge of the jaw and your fingers on the other.

4. Place the tip of the syringe or dropper into the mouth just behind the long canine teeth and push the tip of syringe or dropper slowly into the mouth until it is just past the teeth.

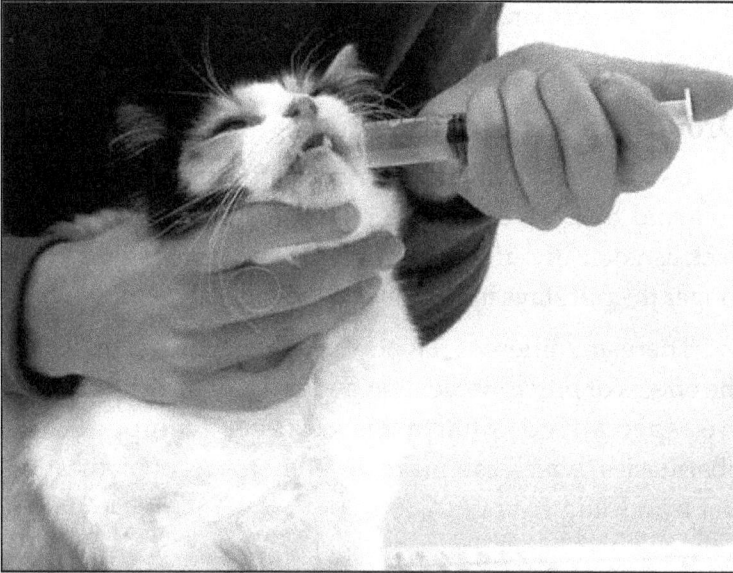

5. Slowly administer the medicine in small amounts with a slight pause between each portion. Do not give it too faster as cat will not be able to swallow it. Never give all of the liquid at once, it may cause choking or vomiting. If your cat spit out some of the medicine, do not re-administer another dose until and unless you feel the cat spit out the entire dose.

6. Hold the cat's mouth closed in a normal position, which will make swallowing easier. Gently rub or blow on your cat's nose as it stimulates a cat to lick her nose and then swallow.

7. Wipe off any medication from your cat's face with a soft, moist cloth.

8. Talk to your cat and give his/her a treat as this will make the next time easier.

9. Finally rinse the syringe or dropper and return the medication to the refrigerator, if necessary.

Drooling After Medication

Usually cats salivate after receiving oral medication. To avoid this, try to put the pill on the base of tongue, as back as you can put, so she will swallow it right away. The longer the pill stays in her mouth, the more she will salivate.

There are different flavors available, which may lessen the effects of bitter medication and reduce salivating. There are specialized pharmacies called 'compounding pharmacies' which can make different forms of medication just by adding flavors.

Chapter 12
Care of Coat

Whatever type of kitten you have, they need to be groomed regularly. It will help you to examine the kitten in detail on a frequent basis. You can check for the presence of fleas and lice and may find some lumps that should be checked by your Vet. The younger your kitten is when you start handling and grooming, the more quickly it will accept the procedure. You can brush your cat, can check its eyes and ears and even can trim its nails. You cannot expect from your semi-grown cat to simply sit for its first grooming session and accept the pulling and cutting without any complaint. So it is necessary to groom your cat regularly since kitten hood.

Grooming Equipments

The extents of grooming kit vary according to the type of kitten you have. If you have a cat with long coat and thick under coat, you will need a number of tools; but for short coat cat, you need very less grooming equipments.

There are many types of brushes available in the market, the most common include:

1. *Bristle brushes:* They can be used on most coat types and vary according to the spacing between bristles and the length of the bristles. The longer the hair coat, the more widely spaced and longer the bristles should be. For the coarser hair coat, you need the stiffer bristles.

2. *Wire-pin Brushes:* These are preferred for medium to long hair and curly or woolly coats.

3. *Slicker brushes:* These brushes have fine wire bristles and are useful for removing mats and tangles.

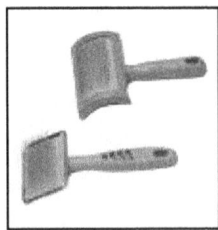

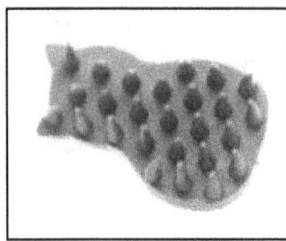

4. *Fine-toothed combs:* They are good to remove small knots of hair.

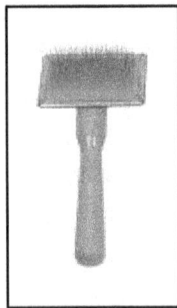

Slicker Brushes   **Rubber Curry Brush**

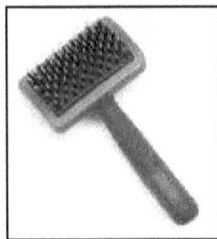

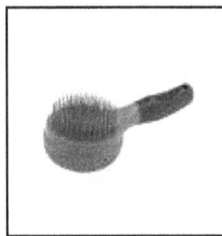

Wire Pin Brushes

5. *Rubber curry brushes:* These are effective at massaging the skin and removing dead hair. They are good to use as a final follow-up to a grooming session.

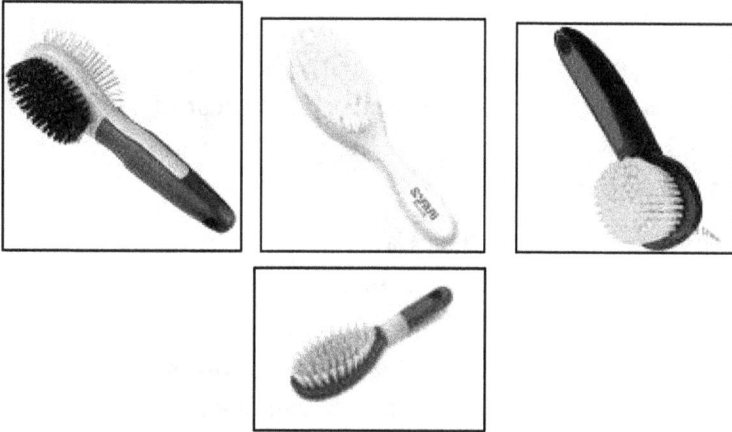

Bristle Brushes

Be gentle during grooming session and be careful while removing mats. The best way to build trust and to make it more pleasurable for both of you is to brush your cat daily.

Brushing and Bathing

You may need to learn the simple procedures about brushing and bathing your cat, to improve your results and make this easier on you and your pet.

Brushing

Brushing should be done to remove all loose hair and for cleaning of the skin. You may use a spray to detangle the mats and to make brushing easier. Brushing should be done systematically *i.e.* start at the head and work towards the tail. Use firm, but gentle strokes. Pulling through tangles and mats may hurt your cat's skin and may lose trust. So take your time to make it a pleasurable experience.

For cats with thick coats, first brush against the grain starting at the skin and brushing outward. When the entire coat is brushed this way, start over and brush with the grain. For other coats, brush with the grain. Always use long strokes for long-haired cats and short strokes for short or wiry hair cats. After brushing, you can use a comb to remove the loose hair.

Grooming a Longhaired Cat

☆ You can use a wide-toothed comb to remove debris and tease out mats. Once the comb runs through the hair, you can change it to a fine-toothed type. Now using a wire brush, remove all dead hair.

☆ Now you can run the fine-toothed comb through the hair in an upward movement, brushing the fur out around the neck so that it forms a ruff.

☆ With the help of a toothbrush, gently brush the shorter hairs on the cat's face. Be careful not to get too close to its eyes.

☆ Finally, you can use the wide-toothed comb to separate the hair and help it to stand up. For show cats, you can use a slicker brush to fluff out the tail.

Grooming a Shorthaired Cat

☆ For such cats, you can use a fine-toothed metal comb, from its head to its tail. As you comb, look for black, shiny specks – a sign of fleas.

☆ Use a rubber brush along the line of the hair. If your cat is rex-coated, this brush is essential as it won't scratch the skin.

☆ With shorthair cat you may prefer to use a soft natural bristle brush, rather than the rubber type.

☆ After brushing and combing, rub the body. This will remove grease from the coat.

Bathing

Before bathing, you should brush your cat. Kitchen sinks or laundry tubs are good for small pets, whereas bathroom tubs are best for larger pets. You must use lukewarm water for the best results.

Insert a cotton ball in the ears to prevent water from entering the canals and apply an ophthalmic ointment to protect the eyes. A variety of shampoos are available in the market; you can choose according to your pet's hair coat, skin condition or specific results. Do not use shampoos made for humans as they contain harsher detergents and not pH balanced for pets and could damage hair or skin.

To give proper bath to your pet, thoroughly soak it and apply the shampoo. Do it in a systematic way *i.e.* from neck to tail, massage the shampoo into the hair and down to the skin. Always use a towel saturated with water and shampoo to wash the face. Rinse the body completely especially groin area, between the toes and armpits. Apply a second application of shampoo if necessary and rinse again.

Drying Off

Squeeze excess water from coat; use a towel to rub the hair first with the grain, then against in a systemic way working from head to tail. Long-haired cats should be combed to prevent tangles while the animal is drying. Do not leave your pet outside, until it is completely dry. For a fluffy appearance to the coat, you can blow dry long-haired cats while brushing hair against the grain. To remove this fluffed appearance, finish by brushing hair with the grain.

Grooming Frequency for Your Cat

Grooming frequency depends on a number of factors including the length of your cat's hair, the ability of the cat to groom herself, the amount of hair shedding and how much it is liked by your cat.

Usually cats with long hair need frequent grooming, often on a daily basis, while cats with short hair can be brushed several times a week. Sick or overweight cats have less ability to groom themselves. Even older cats may have arthritis and also tend to groom less. So these cats should be groomed on a more frequent basis.

Cats do not shed the same amount of hair throughout the year. When your cat is shedding less hair, you may brush or comb your cat and remove very little hair. Whenever your cat is shedding more hair, you need to groom her quite often. It will help in decreasing the risk of developing hairballs. Cats, which love to be groomed, will give you the excellent ways to spend time with them.

Hair Mats

The hair coat gets small tangles in it when left in its natural state. These tangles may get snarled together and the dead hair, debris and shedding hair get caught in the snarl. Whenever brushing or combing is not a routine, these mats become bigger and may become more painful for the animal. Skin can become irritated from the constant pulling. If cat is severely matted, you may need to consult a professional groomer.

Chapter 13
Care of Eyes

Eyes of a healthy cat should be moist and clear. If there is redness or swelling or any discharge from the eye, it indicates infection. If you suspect something wrong, take your cat to the Vet.

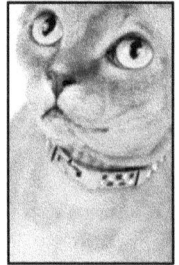

Few guidelines for care of your cat's eyes:

☆ Keep eyes clear of mucus at all times. Always use a sterile eye wash to keep the eye area clean.

☆ Keep all hair out of cat's eyes as hair can cause scratches to the cornea.

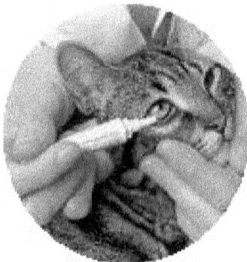
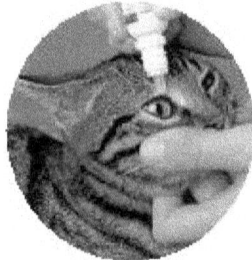

☆ Always apply an ophthalmic ointment under the top lid to protect the eyes before bathing, facial cleanings and insecticide treatment.

☆ Cats with flat faces may have moist eyes always because the fluid is not able to drain away properly through the tear ducts, causing tear staining on the fur at the inner corner of the eyes.

Gently wipe this away with a cotton ball dampened with clean water. Use a separate piece of cotton for each eye and dry with more cotton or a soft tissue.

You can clean hair in affected areas at least weekly with a tear stain remover product.

Chapter 14
Care of Ear

The tissues lining the ear canals are very delicate and easily damaged. I always advise not to tamper with ears at

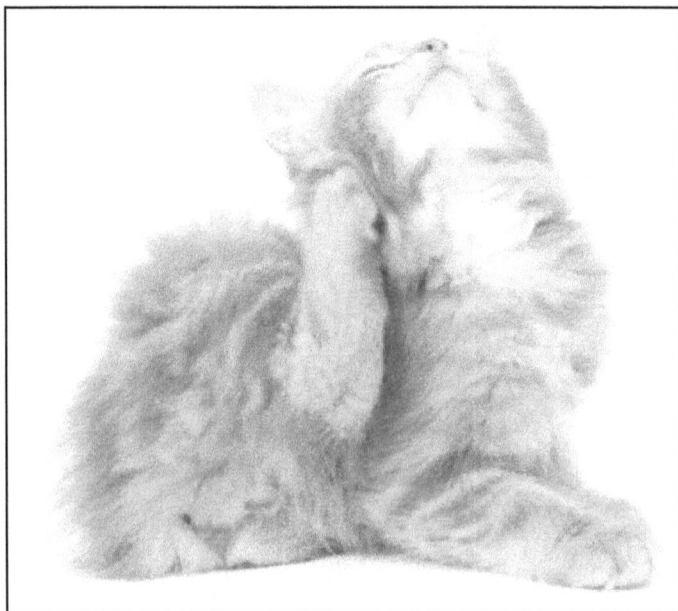

all, however, if you do need to clean the ears, use a cotton ball moistened with oil and just wipe the outer part of the ears with a very light motion. Never poke the cotton into kitten's inner ear.

Ear Disease

Cat's ears may have a terrible odor and may scratch her ears constantly. The ears have dark, crumbly material in them. In such conditions you need to consult your Vet.

Sings of Ear Disease

☆ Odor

☆ Discharge from the ears

☆ Scratching of ears and head

☆ Redness or swelling of the ear canal

☆ Shaking of the head or tilting it to one side

☆ Pain around the ears

☆ Change in behavior of cat

Ear disease is one of the most common conditions. The inflammation of ear canal is called as 'Otitis externa'.

Causes of Ear Disease

The different possible causes are as follows:

(a) Parasites

The ear mite, is a common cause of ear problems especially in kittens. These animals may scratch so severely to traumatize the ear.

(b) Allergies

Cats which are allergic to food or air, may have ear problems. The ear problem may be the first sign of allergy.

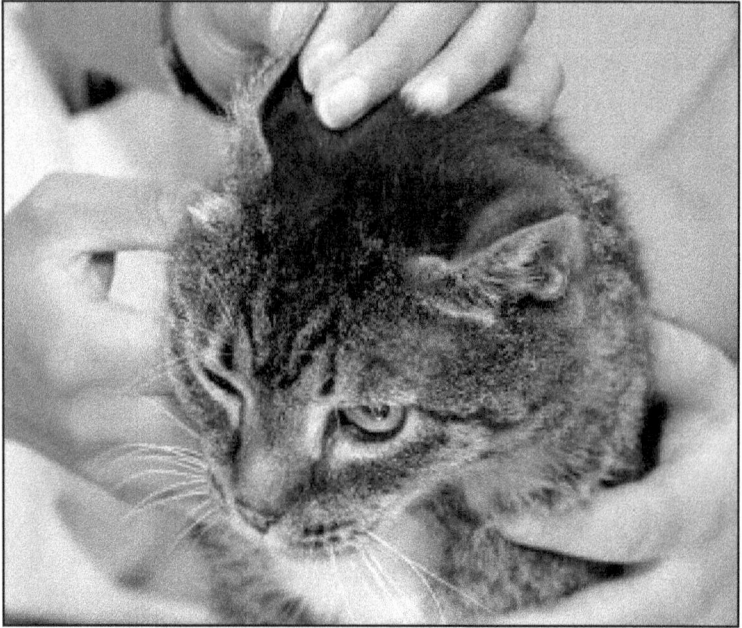

Sometimes we see secondary infections with bacteria or yeast. So along with treating the infection, we need to treat the allergies too.

(c) Bacteria and Yeast

Different types of bacteria and the yeast cause ear infections.

(d) Foreign Bodies

Sometimes plant pawn or cat's fur can enter the ear canal. Due to irritation, the cat scratches a lot and may have traumatized and infected ear. So you must check the ears on routine basis.

(e) Hormonal Imbalance

Deficiency or excess of hormone can result in skin and ear problems.

(f) Other Causes

There are rare hereditary causes which affect the ears. Eosinophilic Granulomas are related to a disorder of the immune system and can occur in the ears of cats.

Diagnosis

Your Vet will check the ear with the help of an otoscope. Swabs of the ear can be taken, smeared on a microscope slide, stained and examined for bacteria, yeast and mites. A thorough examination may help determine if this could be hormonal, allergic or hereditary problem. If bacterial infection does not respond to the first antibiotic therapy, a culture and sensitivity may need to be performed to select a different antibiotic.

Treatment

Always consult your Vet for proper diagnosis and treatment.

How to Clean Ears

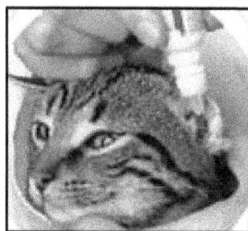

Cat's ear is more L-shaped than yours, and debris loves to collect at the corner of the L. To remove this debris, fill your cat's ear canal with a good ear cleaner. Ear cleaners should be slightly acidic but should not sting. Massage the base of the ear for 20-30 seconds to soften and release the debris. Wipe out the loose debris and excess fluid with a cotton ball. Repeat the procedure until you see no more debris.

Cotton swabs can be used to clean the inside of the earflap and the part of the ear canal you can see. Do not go further down in the ear canal since that tends to pack debris in the ear canal, rather than removing it.

Some of the ear problems are so painful; the cat must be anesthetized to do a good job of cleaning the ears.

After the ear is clean, let the cat shake her head and allow sometime for the ears to dry.

Prevention

The key to healthy ears is to keep them clean. Check your cat's ears weekly. Treat any underlying condition that predisposes your cat to ear problems.

If the cat is in severe discomfort, the ears have a bad smell, do not delay in contacting your Vet.

Chapter 15
Dental Care

Brushing your teeth should be an enjoyable time for both of you. If you take things slowly at the beginning and give lots of praise to your cat, it will make brushing session easier for both of you.

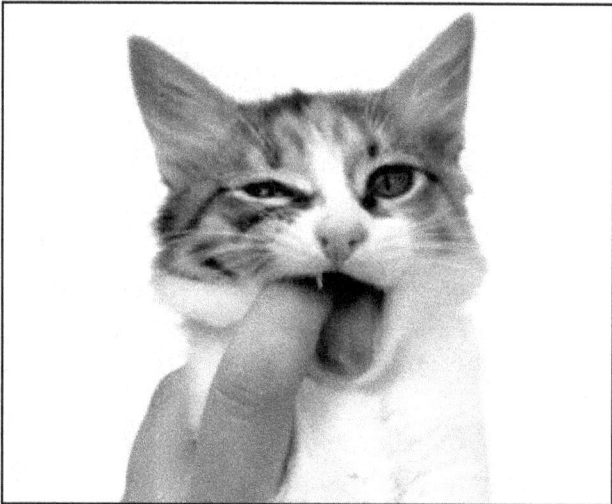

Toothpaste

There are so many pet toothpastes available in the market. Human toothpastes can upset cat's stomach. Cat toothpastes contain several different active ingredients and flavored toothpastes can make tooth brushing more acceptable to pets.

Toothbrushes, Sponges

The exact benefit of tooth brushing comes from the mechanical action of the brush on the teeth. Different brushes, sponges and pads are available. The choice depends on the health of your cat's gums, your ability to clean the teeth and the cooperation of your cat. Usually tooth brushes designed for cats are smaller, ultra-soft and of different shape. Finger tooth brushes do not have a handle, but fit over your finger. For some cats dental sponges or pads are helpful as they are more pliable, softer than brushes and are disposable.

How to Brush

Brushing sessions should be short and positive. Do not overly restrain your cat and be sure to praise your cat throughout the process.

1. Firstly, have your cat get used to you putting things in her mouth. Dip your finger in tuna water, chicken or meat broth or other liquid your cat may like. Call your cat with a voice "treat" and let your cat lick the liquid off your finger. Now rub your soaked finger gently over your cat's gums and teeth. Repeat it for few times till your

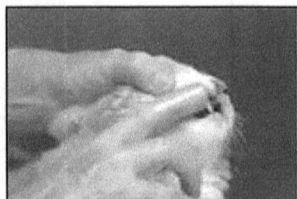

cat actually look forward to this and you can move on.

2. Now place gauze around your finger and you can dip it in tuna water or other liquid. Gently rub the teeth in circular motion with your gauzed finger. Repeat this for a number of times and let your cat will feel comfortable with this procedure. Do not forget to praise her during and after the procedure.

3. When your cat gets used to have flavored gauze in her mouth, you can start using tooth brush or pad. Your cat should get used to the consistency of these items. Let your cat lick something tasty

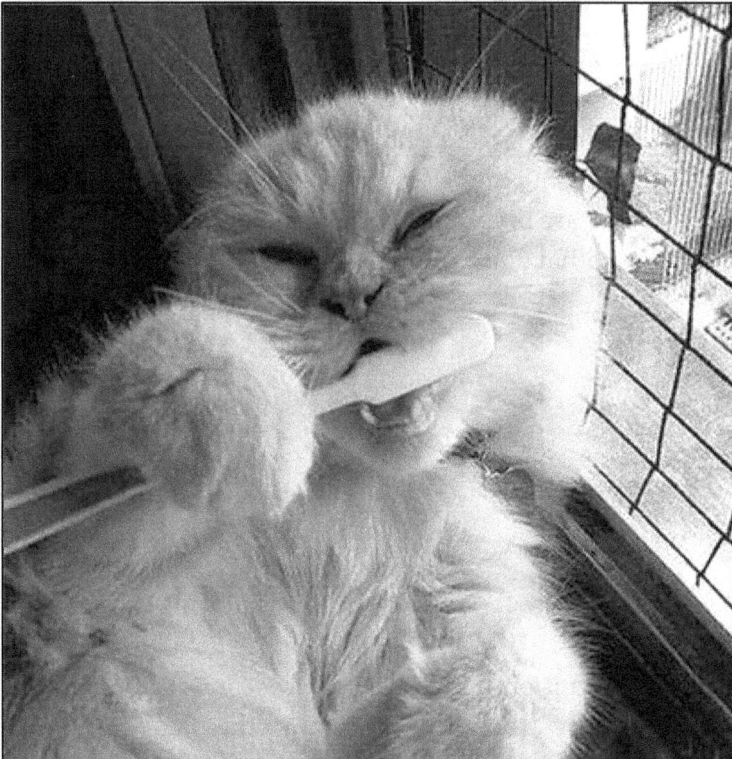

from the brush or pad, so she gets used to the texture.

4. Once the cat is used to the cleaning item, you can add the toothpaste. Get your cat used to the flavor and consistency of the tooth paste. Praise your cat always.

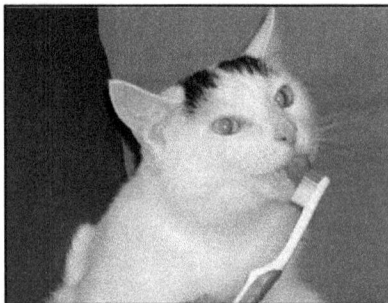

5. Now you are ready to start brushing. Talk to your cat in a happy voice during the process and praise your cat at the end. At first start brushing with one tooth and slowly increase the number of teeth you are brushing. Try to make it a game; you both will have fun doing it.

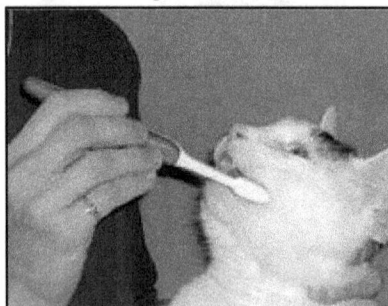

Frequency of Brushing

Try to do it on daily basis. If you cannot brush daily, brushing every other day will remove the plaque.

Chapter 16
Hairballs

Hairballs are an ever-present problem which to some degree can be forestalled by regular grooming of the coat as it is shed to make way for the new growth. Shedding goes on practically all the time, though it is more evident in spring, summer and fall. The loosening of the old hair makes him uncomfortable; he rubs himself along the carpet in an effort to get rid of it. Out of doors he rolls on the grass.

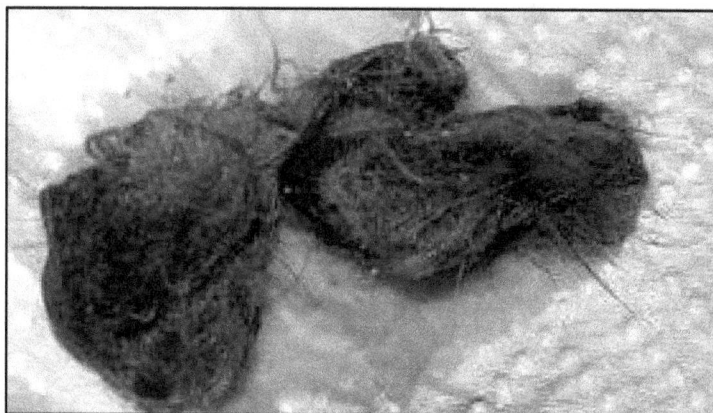

Indoors he licks his forefeet, and then uses them like hand to rub his face and body, meantime ingesting the shedding hair.

He swallows a considerable amount of hair that forms mats and ropes in stomach and intestines to interfere with adequate elimination and in severe cases to cause death. Retching, coughing, vomiting and constipation may be due to hairball obstruction. Prevention is better than cure though often both are needed. You can give a teaspoonful of olive oil or mineral oil or white Vaseline every week when shedding is evident. If your cat objects to forcible medication, you can add the oil to his favorite food. Do not use castor oil like strong purgatives for hairball treatment, as they can be harmful to your cat.

Chapter 17
Clipping Nails

Clipping your cat's nail is not just a part of grooming, but is important for its health as well. The untrimmed nails can lead to a variety of problems like broken nails that are painful and can bleed. The unclipped nails can get caught in the carpet, clothes or furniture.

How many owners put off trimming cat's nails until the Veterinary check-up comes around and the Veterinarian must do it? Many cat owners may be hesitant to trim their cat's nails because they are afraid of cutting the quick of the nail, which may cause pain or bleeding.

While trimming your cat's nails, you are only cutting away the excess. Now you need to know what is excess

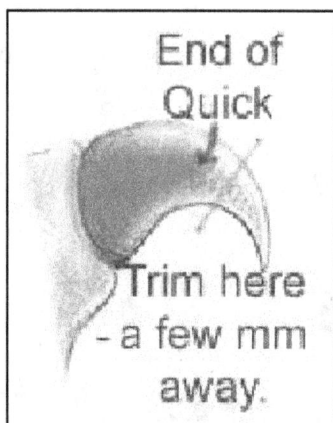

End of Quick

Trim here - a few mm away.

and how to make nail trimming a painless process for both you and your cat.

Procedure

You will need a high quality pair of trimmers, some styptic powder, and styptic pads to stop bleeding if you nick the quick.

1. You may sit on the floor with your cat, hold your cat in your lap or have someone hold your cat on a table. Hold your cat's paw firmly and push on her pads to extend the nail. Locate where the quick ends with clear or light nails, it is easy to see the pink color where the quick ends.

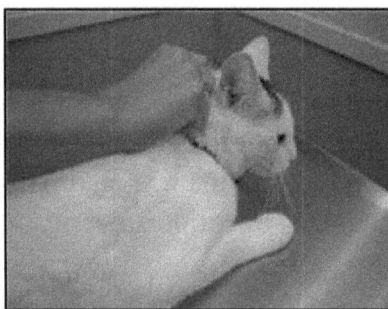

2. With the help of a nail trimmer for cats, cut the nails below the quick on a 45 degree angle, with the cutting end of the nail clipper toward the end

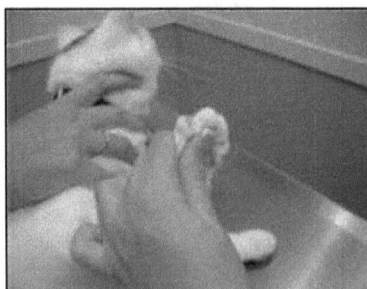

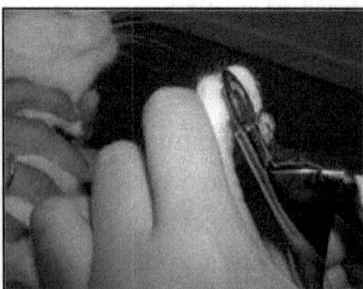

of the nail. In cats, quick is very easy to see and you can cut the excess away with one cut.

3. If the nails are brittle, the cut may tend to splinter the nail. In such cases, file the nail in a sweeping motion starting from the back of the nail and following the curve to the tip.

4. If the cat is comfortable during the procedure, do all four feet. If she is not, take a break. Do not forget the dewclaws. If not trimmed, dewclaws can grow so long they curl up, grow into soft tissue like a painful ingrown toe nail.

5. If you accidentally cut the quick, wipe off the blood and apply styptic powder to check bleeding. It is not serious and will heal in a very short time.

Tips

It is better to trim a small amount on a regular basis. Always buy a good pair of nail trimmers as it will last a lifetime.

Chapter 18
Feeding

Feeding the cat today is less of a chore than it has ever been before, a fact that without doubt has served as an additional incentive to an ever-growing number of people who keep a cat as pet and companion. Before you consider exactly what you would like to feed, it is therefore worth taking a moment or two to learn about your kitten's special nutritional requirements.

Increasing knowledge of the science of nutrition has enabled manufacturers to prepare diets with the ingredients which are balanced for cats of all ages *i.e.* for growth, maintenance and lactation. These foods are readily available in cans and packages for instant feeding.

Cats are efficient hunters and they cannot rely on vegetarian food as a source of nutrition. However, they need some specific nutrients found only in animal tissues like Vitamin A and Niacin. They also need high level of dietary protein, as the amino-acid taurine is vital for a cat's eyesight and it cannot be manufactured from other materials. Cats are known as "obligate carnivores"- they cannot live on a vegetarian diet and must eat meat.

Type of Food

1. Commercial Foods

This category has two types of foods.

(a) Canned Food

A wide variety of canned foods are available in the market   which include beef, lamb, chicken, liver, tuna fish etc. These foods are available on cheaper and costlier prices. Cheaper canned foods usually contain maximum portion of cereals which are not useful for cat, while costlier canned foods contain proper concentration of meat or chicken or fish. You should always note the ingredients to know the nutritive value of the product and level of Vitamin B as it gets easily destroyed due to heat.

(b) Dry Foods

These are packaged as broken, fine-kibbled and granular   food and are available in different flavors containing meat or fish or chicken and fat, vitamins, cereals and other preservatives. These foods are well balanced foods to meet the cat's requirement.

2. Milk

Milk has been called the cat's best friend. The calcium component of milk is vital. It is needed for bones and teeth, blood clotting, body fluids and soft tissues.

Whole milk is very nutritious. Dried skim milk contains all the solids and minerals but lacks fat which incorporate the fat-soluble Vitamin –A. So it will be useful to add whole milk to it.

Usually cats and weaned kittens do not require milk as part of their diet and certainly not as a substitute for water. Some cats cannot digest lactose, a sugar found in milk and can have stomach upsets. Such cats should not be fed with milk.

3. Eggs

Eggs are known as nature's storehouse and are suitable for cats of any age. The egg yolk is superior to the white as a source of minerals, fats and vitamins. The egg white is egg protein. The yolk can be fed raw or cooked whereas the white is not readily digestible in raw form. The egg white should not be fed in excess as it may inhibit the absorption of Vitamin B2 (Biotin).

4. Meat

The animal proteins *i.e.* meat and fish, constitute the mainstay of the daily diet. Proteins build the bony structure, hence are vital for maximum growth and development. Practically all kinds of meat are suitable – beef, lamb, chicken, horse meat and rabbit. Meat should be kept at adequate refrigeration temperature for storage. Once thawed, it must be fed at once. Raw meat can be baked or steamed to prevent the natural juices. Liver is very good for cats but excess feeding will cause diarrhea. Likely lungs and spleen may also cause diarrhea.

5. Chicken

This can be given in cooked form. Even rabbits can also be fed to cats in raw or cooked form. Precautions should be taken not to feed bones as their sharp edges can cause internal damage.

6. Fish

Salt-water fish, valuable for its iodine content, is also enjoyed as an alternate to meat. Fresh fish should never be fed raw as it commonly harbors dangerous parasites. Cook it well and before serving and finger it carefully to remove bones, as they are harmful to the cat. Canned tuna, salmon and shrimp are well-known favorites which of course, require no cooking.

7. Broths

Broth in which meat has been cooked is valuable as a moistener for broken biscuit or meal and as a conveyor for vegetables which the pet might otherwise not take willingly. The food value of broth may be increased if the meat is plunged into cold water and then simmered for an hour or two. Cold water draws out the extractives from the meat into the broth, whereas boiling water tends to seal the pores and hold the juices more nearly within the piece.

8. Vegetables

Vegetables are usually not relished by the cat unless accompanied by meat or fish. String beans and peas are probably the most nourishing, while spinach, carrots and tomatoes are superior in Vitamin content. Cooked vegetables are apt to be more easily digested than raw vegetables, though their vitamin content may be impaired by heat. The tomato is in a class by itself; it is just as vitamin-filled and as easy to digest raw as when cooked.

9. Cereals

While vegetables do contain a certain amount of carbohydrates, the latter are furnished principally by the cereals – barely, rice, wheat, bread and so on. Rice and barely should be steamed to a pulp. Wheat can be provided by whole wheat kinds.

Although the starches should compromise only a small proportion of the daily diet, they are valuable when incorporated in food mixtures in that they are needed in conjunction with the fats.

10. Grass

Usually they use tough-fibered grass as an emetic when he feels uncomfortable from overeating or from eating something distasteful. Don't worry about it. It is an instinctive act about which the pet doubtless knows best.

Amount of Food

Cats are more naturally "snackers" and will eat 10 to 20 small meals a day. If you give your kitten dry food on a "free-choice" basis, you will notice it returning to the bowl many times during the day for a quick snack, rather than working its way through the food at one sitting. Cats fed on moist food do tend to eat bigger meals, but most would probably prefer small and frequent meals to one large bowlful given at the end of the day. Cats often do not let us get away with infrequent feeding and demand more every time you go into the kitchen.

A kitten needs small, frequent meals in order to be able to ingest and digest enough nutrients to grow rapidly and must be fed much more frequently than an adult cat. When you first get your kitten at 8 to 12 weeks of age, it will need about five meals a day. If you are out during the day time, one way to manage this is to provide dry food, which can be left for the kitten to help itself as it likes. When the kitten is six months old and about 75 percent of its full size, you can reduce meal times to twice a day.

Where to Feed

You should feed your kitten in a quiet spot where there will be no competition from other cats and no chance of the food being stolen by a dog, and where there will be no other interruptions. Be sure to place your kitten's feeding bowl away from its litter box.

Water: If you feed your kitten on a canned moist food, it may not drink water because most of the water if requires will be provided by the food. An average adult cat requires a minimum of about 150 ml of water per day. As one cannot know exactly how much your kitten is taking in with its food, you must always keep a supply of clean and fresh water so that kitten can adjust its intake to suit itself.

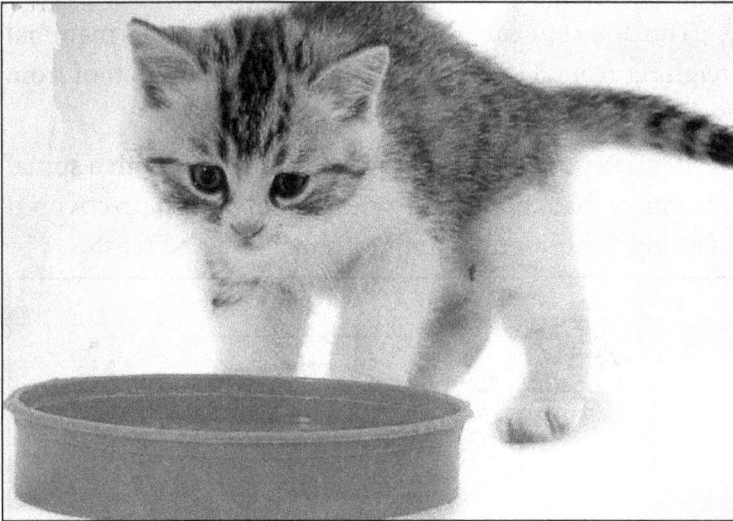

Chapter 19
Anatomy of a Cat

The domestic cat is a digitigrades, carnivorous mammal weighing from 3 to 8 kg, with an average life span of from twelve to fourteen years.

It is categorized as a vertebrate animal *i.e.* with a spinal column or backbone and whose multiple hair-covered offspring feed upon the milk of the mother's breasts.

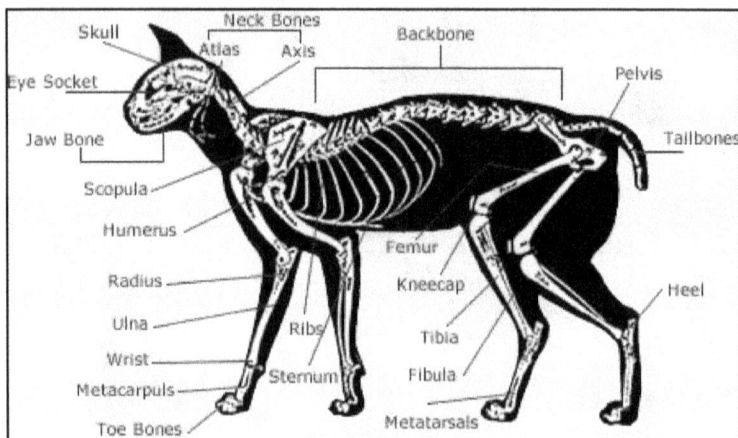

Cat's Skeletal System

Carnivorous animals are flesh-eating mammals. These animals have canine teeth, two in each jaw, designed for ripping and tearing the flesh of their captured prey.

The term digitigrades refers to the posture of the food. The digitigrades foot walks and runs on its toes with the heel up in the air, as opposed to the plantigrade good that plants its entire sole from toes to heel flat on the ground.

The cat does not have great speed as a ground runner. Instead, stealth and jumping ability compensated for lack of endurance in the chase. The cat's hind legs are a bit longer than his forelegs; they are stronger and limber as a coiled spring.

Cat's body is longer than its approximate eight-inch height. The leg muscles are very well developed, strong, flexible and practically fashioned for jumping and climbing. These qualities are accompanied by a remarkable degree of balance and coordination. In the event of a fall, the cat can literally turn himself in the air so as to land on all fours. But it's not always true; in fact cats can die by falling from a height.

The tail also plays some part in contributing to balance, although coordination is governed to greater extent by the inner ear. Mostly the tail is long, rounded and fur-covered to its tip. The cat swings its tail slowly and gracefully except in anger when its pace is considerably increased.

The toes-five on the forefeet, four on the hind feet – are thickly cushioned so the cat can move along without making a sound. The soles are not tough and are easily irritated by prolonged running on rough terrain.

The claws–The cat's claws are retractile and are capable of being completely sheathed or extended as conditions

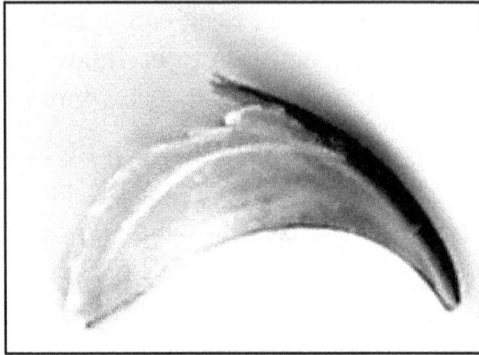

Cat's Claw

warrant. When the animal is at rest and undisturbed, the claws are drawn back into a sheath. When needed for climbing, fighting or capturing prey, they are drawn forward and downward by an elastic tendon. When exposed, they are sharp as little knives. These claws are the cat's only defensive weapon.

'Kneading' - The claws can be extended or contracted at will; it is known as kneading. It can be observed in nursing kittens when they knead the mother's breast as if to help to stimulate the milk flow. In later life when accompanied by purring, kneading seems to furnish an emotional outlet indicating pleasure or contentment.

The wild cat clawed tree trunks to manicure his nails and incidentally strengthen his muscles; the domestic cat today uses the scratching post for the same purpose.

The teeth–There are two sets of teeth – temporary or milk teeth and the permanent teeth which erupt at about five months of age. The permanent teeth are adapted for cutting and tearing rather than for crushing and grinding.

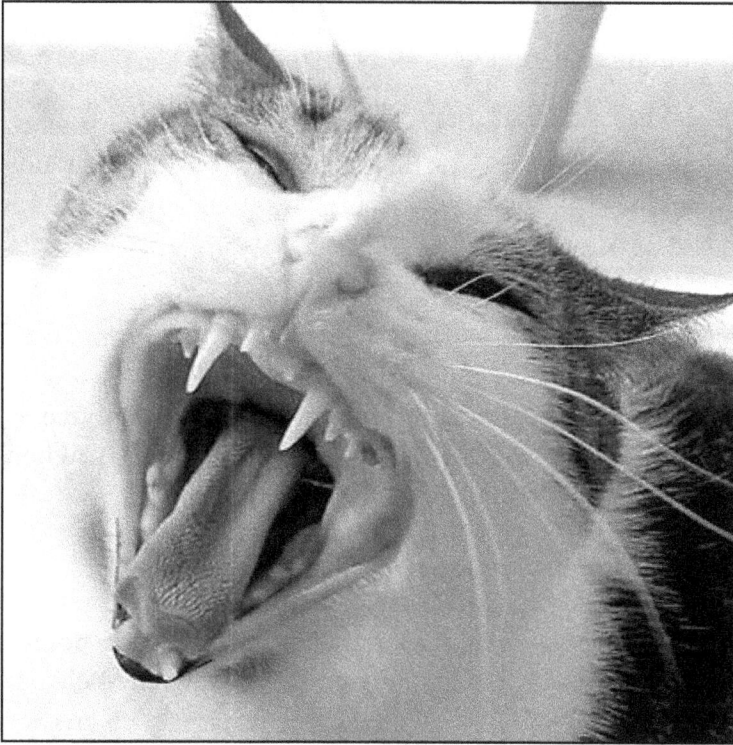

Directly in front of each jaw are six small incisors; flanked by the larger canine teeth, one upper and one lower on each side. Then three premolars on each side in the upper jaw and two in the lower jaw and behind them one molar on each side in each jaw. This entire set of thirty permanent teeth is usually complete at eight months of age.

The teeth should be regularly inspected since they are subject to tartar accumulation and pyorrhea. Removal of tartar is a tricky business to the Veterinarian lest the tender gums be lacerated in the process. Decay with or without ulceration is unusual, but when it does occur it can cause such pain that the animal refuse to eat. Brushing the teeth with tooth paste on regular basis may help to preserve them to a good old age.

Whiskers and Tongue

The whiskers and the tongue may be considered as aids to stalking. They help him feel his way along when he hunts in the dark and cannot see.

Rough surface tongue serves as brush and comb. He uses it consistently to clean his coat and at the same time pull out loose hairs about to be shed. Persistent licking of the coat may be an instinctive act designed to remove as much as possible if the cat's body scent so that, when stalking, he will not alert his victims to his presence.

Sense of Smell

The sense of smell is acute enough to track prey for short distances. Stealth and patience are its strong points. He prefers to sit for hours, if needed, beside a tiny hole out of which he/she knows by the scent that a rat will emerge sooner or later. The moment it does, he springs on it like lightening, biting it or stunning it with a blow of his paws. The average cat does not kill to eat; just for fun he captures almost any small thing that moves whether it be a rat or a mouse or a bug.

A cat's scenting is at its best when the nose is cool and moist since moisture enhances scenting ability. An indoor cat especially may have a warm nose simply because he lives in a warm house. A hot, dry nose may indicate a feverish condition.

Sense of Hearing

The cat's hearing is also acute except in all white cats which may be congenitally deaf. The normal cat can detect sounds so slight as to be unnoticed by human beings. Comparatively small, the ears are set wide on top of the skull, carried stiffly erect and are tilted slightly outward and forward. Fine hairs within the cup of the ear screen out particles of foreign matter; even so, the ears do collect a certain amount of dust and dirt as well as an accumulation of wax.

Ear mites, such tiny parasites that you never notice them, frequently infest the ears and promote intolerable itching. Canker, an ulcerous and not infrequent ear condition, can become very serious if not expertly treated. The best way is to inspect the ears daily, to keep them clean and to regard persistent scratching as a signal for immediate action.

Sense of Sight

As compared with body size, the eyes are large. Placed wide apart and well to the front, their vision is binocular *i.e.* both eyes see the image at the same time. All newborn kittens have blue eyes which occasionally with growth darken to a deeper shade, or they may end up at maturity as hazel, orange, brown, green or yellow. The cat sees best in dim light but he cannot see in total darkness. The cat cannot detect color and is either totally or partially color blind. These animals can distinguish degree of luminosity or brightness indistinguishable to the human eye.

The eyes are a good indicator of health. They should appear bright, clean, clear and wide open. A bit of yellowish matter in the corners needs to be considered serious. Eyes red and weeping with sticky matter may indicate a subnormal condition resulting from Vitamins deficiency or otherwise improper feeding and which requires medication.

Coat and Skin

The cat's coat is often his best bid for popular favor. It is thing of beauty, unusual colors which include white, black, blue silver, red, cream, brown, and smoke and so on. It may be spotted, banned or ticked in pattern.

The skin of the healthy cat is elastic and loose-fitting, and the coat is so luxuriant that the animal seldom if ever needs a man-made coat.

Shedding goes on practically all the time, though it is more noticeable when the coat is being prepared by nature for the temperature of the season just ahead. The old coat is apt to be lifeless and a bit faded; the new growth is bright, shining and more accurately intense in its color.

Chapter 20
Going on Vacation

Many owners are worried about the welfare of their cats or kittens while they are away. That's the reason they do not fully enjoy their annual vacations. But if you plan everything with little organization and research, you will be able to find a good solution and to go for a nice vacation. You may have following options to leave your kitten in good hands.

Leaving Your Kitten with a Neighbor

Leaving a kitten alone in the house, with a neighbor coming in to feed and check on it – even just for two or three days – is not a very good idea. Kittens are mischief in nature, especially if they are bored. So it's better to arrange for a friend to stay in your house, this would be preferable to popping in once or even twice a day.

The kitten should not be allowed outdoors, as caring for another person's pet is a great responsibility and even a temporary disappearance of your kitten would be upsetting for you and the person left in charge. It will be better to provide an indoor litter box for the kitten to use and be sure to leave full instructions regarding food, water, medications and play. An older kitten or cat that is used to being alone will be safe for a day or two. The younger the cat, the more advisable it is to keep it indoors for the short period when you are going to be away.

Before going for vacation, give details of where to contact you in an emergency, address and telephone number of your Veterinary clinic to the person. It is also a good idea to inform your Vet that you will be away. If the person is not familiar with area, it will be helpful if you draw a road map of how to get the clinic.

Boarding Kennel

If you are going away for more than a few days, the best way to ensure your kitten's health and safety is to choose a good boarding kennel. You can ask your Vet for recommendation in your area or can check with your friends or neighbors for boarding kennels.

You need to know that your kitten will be safe and properly fed, you also want a kennel to be run by staff who will spend time with the kitten and make it feel at home *i.e.*, to care for it as you do. The place should be clean and hygienic. You must consider the following points to help you choose the best kennel for your kitten:

(*a*) Cleanliness

If the kennel owner does not give you a tour, look elsewhere. The reason is very much practical and logical as the owner of a good kennel will be pleased to let you see how it is run and where your kitten will be kept.

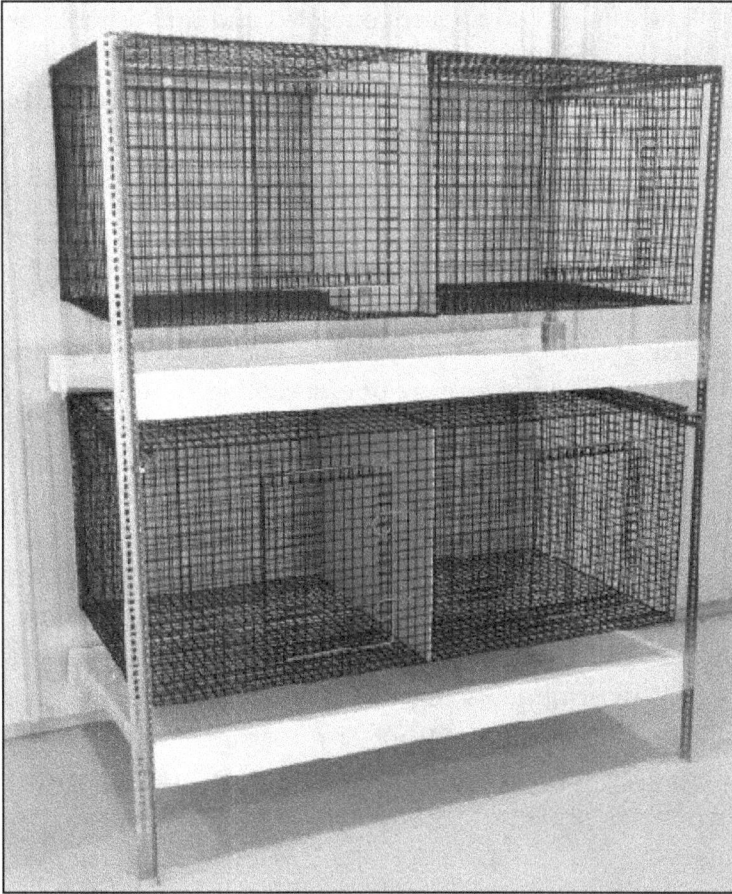

Look for clean, well-kept premises in tidy and well-tended surroundings. The building should be well maintained and the enclosures and their concrete bases should be free of algae stains. The place should have an individual open-air exercise area and a comfortable sleeping area. The best kennels will not only take care to keep your cat in clean and safe conditions, but also keep them occupied and have something interesting to look at.

The cats should appear contented and there should be no obvious smell in their environment, either of feces and urine or of strong disinfectant. Water bowls should be clean and filled with fresh water, food bowls should also clean properly and the food provided should be fresh and suitable to each cat.

Litter boxes should be clean and sufficiently large for the cats to use. Make sure to check for type of litter used and ask about how frequently the litter is changed. Check for the provision of heating or of a cooling system.

(b) Minimizing Infections

The kennel should insist that your kitten has been fully vaccinated against feline panleukopenia infection, cat flu and they must check for whether primary or booster injections have been carried out far enough in advance to allow maximum protection and should check that cat have been dewormed on regular basis. This should be a fundamental requirement for any boarding kennel. Many cats carry latent health problem that may manifest themselves under stress and can be transmitted to other cats.

(c) Caring Proprietors

A good guide to assess the caring nature of proprietor is whether he or she asks you about your kitten's or cat's medical history and checks that vaccinations are up to date you should also find out whether the kennel would be prepared to continue with any ongoing medication prescribed for the kitten by your Vet.

There are some reported instances in which owners have been given the wrong cat to take home, or have returned to collect their beloved cat only to find that it has disappeared or even worse – has died. However, escape through negligence and death through accident should never be allowed to happen.

When you leave your kitten at the kennel, be sure that the kennel owner knows how to contact you in an emergency and has the details for your Veterinary clinic. Find out what would happen if your kitten were sick while you are on vacation or if you were unable for any reason to collect it on the pre-arranged date.

(d) Timings

You should check with them about admit and pick up hours. What if your return is delayed? You must ask them regarding a time when you can call to check on how your cat is doing.

Chapter 21
Traveling and Shipping

Taking the cat along on a journey can be easy or difficult. It all depends upon whether traveling is a new experience or merely another way of getting around for which the pet has been trained. The trip may be long or short; the conveyance may be a car, a train or somebody's own two feet. Whichever it is, preparation for the journey is very much the same if the cat is not to be frightened out of his wits and owner become so exasperated that he says never again.

Frequent or at least occasional trips to the Veterinarian are also no rarity. Once upon a time the Vet came to the house to treat the ailing cat, but nowadays his patients must visit his clinic for diagnostic facilities. And whether the cat is sick or well, one's arms cannot constitute safe control for the pet of any age or in any state of health.

The Carrier -You can get either a bag or a durable carrier of suitable size, ventilated at one or both ends and covered over the top and secured by strong latches and a strap. The plastic carriers can be cleaned easily and are easy to carry and handle. You can put a towel or blanket or newspapers at the floor of bag or carrier. To the handle attach a label marked with your name and address and the cat's name as well.

The next step is to accustom the pet to the carrier. Let him sleep in it if he likes, or allow him to use it for occasional naps during the day, with the cover alternately laid back or closed, latched and strapped. Begin this training as early in life as possible so the kitten will accept it as just another place in which to relax.

Get him used to being carried around in the bag, first in the house, then around the block and finally in the car. Talk to him as you go, let him see through the screened end and in no time at all he will learn that this is a comfortable way to be moved about. Once thoroughly trained to his own carrier, he gets there in as good condition as when he left home.

When you have plenty of time to prepare for the journey, be sure the claws are clipped to avoid possibility of catching them in the blanket or towel. Do not feed for several hours prior to the take off and give only a small amount of something easily digestible. A few cats are poor travelers in

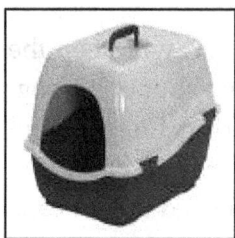

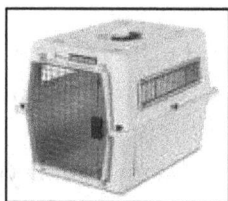

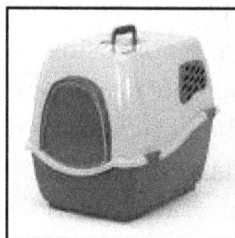

Cat Carriers

spite of all we can do to help them. Sedatives are often advised in such cases but they should not be given except when prescribed by the Veterinarian.

These days few products are available in the market which contains pheromones. These pheromones have calming effects on cats. When these are sprayed into a cat carrier at least half an hour before putting the cat inside, it can have a calming effect on the cat.

Traveling by Car

The majority of cats do not have any problem while car ride. But few timid ones can have some problems and they need to be taught to ride and it is a good idea to give them slow and sensible training. You should stop often on long trips to allow cat to get exercise outside of their crates and to relieve themselves. It is advisable to restrain your cat during traveling in a wire cage or plastic cage. One most important point is to never leave your cat in a hot car. Pets are unable to control their own body temperature and few minutes' exposure to heat can be dangerous to cause irreversible damage or death.

In Hotels and Cottages

Always inform the staff at hotels about your cat and check for the provision to keep them there. When you stop at hotels the carrier is invaluable as a safe sleeping place. A cage, collapsible for easy packing in the car, will keep the pet safe against escape. Furthermore, when shut in his bag, the cat cannot amuse himself manicuring his nails by clawing furniture and draperies. If you stop to eat at the wayside, take the carrier with you. If you need to leave the pet alone in the car, be sure to park in a well shaded area.

On the Train

Ordinarily the cat is allowed to accompany his owner on trains, in compartments when suitably confined to the carrier. Otherwise he will be relegated to the baggage car. If the journey involves more than 24 hours, the cat is better off in the baggage car where the owner is permitted to visit him frequently. For this purpose there are available light weight crates fitted with handles for carrying. They are longer than the average hand held carrier, large enough in fact for the cat to stand up and stretch as well as to turn around and lie down in position. Feeding is not necessary for short trips, although small meal will be enjoyed when the owner makes periodic check on the little traveler.

Shipping

Avoid shipping toward the end of the week and also avoid trips during very cold or very hot weather. Arrange for the trip in advance, first with your Veterinarian regarding the possibility of quarantine restrictions which might prevent the shipment from crossing state lines. Also have your Veterinarian examine the cat thoroughly prior to the start. He will give you a health certificate, which will

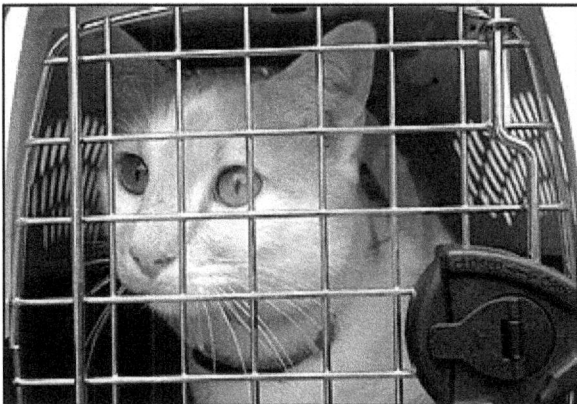

be helpful for future reference in case of accident, neglect or sickness. Try to arrange the journey with a minimum of connections and stops. When plans are completed, send the details of departure and arrival to the new owner.

You must use well ventilated and spacious crates for shipment. The containers for food and water and directions can be attached to the crate. Despite every precaution, shipping a cat has its element of risk. In short, do not ship unless it cannot be avoided.

By Plane

You may want to consider having a boarding facility to take care of your pet while you are away as air travel can be difficult for your pet. Still, if you are going to take your pet, the following guidelines will help you to arrive safely at your destination.

☆ You need to obtain a health certificate from your Veterinarian. This certificate should meet the requirements of your nation of destination and your airline carrier. But there is always a time limit for the certificate. So, you must check this with guidelines.

☆ Always carry the health certificate and your pet's vaccination certificate with you. In some nations, your pet will need to be quarantined at your destination. So, you may need to reconsider the things.

☆ Sedatives and tranquilizers can be used only under the recommendation of your Veterinarian.

☆ Your cat must have an accurate identification tag with complete information including destination address, phone number, and rabies vaccination tag.

Place this information on the outside and inside the crate.

☆ Attach a food and a water dish to the inside of the crate and place them in such a fashion that they can be filled from outside without opening the crate. Also attach a bag of food and a water bottle to the outside of the crate.

☆ Give him food and water within four hours intervals of departure. Always pack a first aid kit for your pet and print "LIVE ANIMAL" on the top and sides of the crate.

☆ Be sure your pet is crate trained and help your pet become accustomed to loud and unfamiliar noises.

☆ Provide plenty of exercise before departure. Book on direct, non-stop flights. Try to travel on the same flight as your pet.

Cold Weather

In cold weather, hypothermia (decrease in body temperature) is a major concern. Inadequate housing, food or becoming wet can make a pet more susceptible to such condition. There are other additional hazards associated with cold weather and the following guidelines will help you to make your cat comfortable and safe in cold weather.

(a) Outdoor Housing

For an outside cat, provide shelter at a place away from the wind. Try to make a small warm area, preferably a crate or box and cover it with warm blanket. Shivering is usually a sign that your pet is too cold and indicates the hypothermia. In such conditions, pet should be warmed slowly till the temperature is normal. These pets will need extra calories to keep them warm. When the temperature is below freezing, you may need to provide extra calories.

Always provide fresh, unfrozen water to your pet. Avoid stainless steel or metal bowls.

Hazards to Outdoor Cat

The cat owners usually keep their pet safe, happy and healthy by setting the following priorities:

- ☆ By keeping their cats indoors
- ☆ By enjoying the outdoors with their pet in shared activity.
- ☆ By creating safe enclosures for unsupervised outdoor activity.

A cat need to play, exercise, rest, good diet and companionship and she can get all these indoors or outdoors. You can make the indoors more appealing for your cat as there are a number of outdoor dangers your cat may face.

Most common outside hazards include:

- ☆ *Accidents*: An outside cat may be hit by a car, which can be life threatening.
- ☆ *Fights:* Your cat may get in to a territorial fight with another cat and could result into painful lumps or an abscess. In such cases take it to the Vet for proper Veterinary care.
- ☆ *Injuries*: Cats can get life threatening injuries from dogs and may need Veterinary attention.
- ☆ *Cruelty*: All people are not cat lovers. There are reports in which cats have been injured by angry neighbors.

☆ *Parasites*: Outdoors cats may pick up fleas, ticks, worms etc.

☆ *Poisons*: Outdoor cats are at risky state of getting exposed to toxic chemicals or poisons.

☆ *Getting lost*: Your cat may be stolen, adopted by others or taken to an animal shelter. So make sure to keep identification on your cat at all times.

How to Make the Outdoors Safer?

☆ *Identification*: Make sure that your cat has a harness or collar with identification tag. Micro-chipping is another alternative.

☆ *Health measures*: Get your cat fully vaccinated, and spayed or neutered. Keep its deworming up to date.

☆ *Door*: Install a cat door connected to a screened-in porch or fence yard, so that your cat may enjoy the outdoors as he desires and provides a quick escape from predators.

☆ *Leash*: You must teach your cat to walk on a leash. It is good to use a retractable lead which will eliminate tugging, pulling and straining. It is best to use a harness instead of a collar in cats.

☆ *Environmental safety*: You can attach a bell to your cat's harness collar to prevent her from attack by other mammals or to alert people that he/she is around.

☆ *Timings*: You can allow your cat outside confined, when you are home and preferably during the day time to reduce the hazards.

Chapter 22
Understanding your Cat

Cat is a fundamentally different animal to you, with its own set of motivations, attitudes and social behavior.

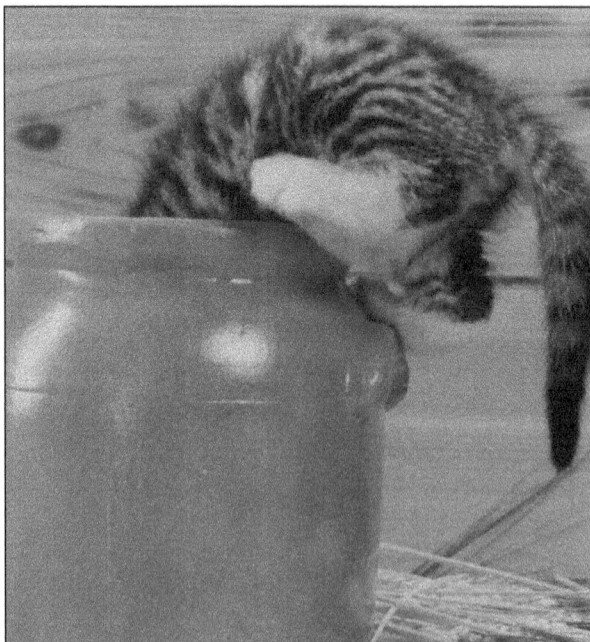

1. Intelligence and Awareness

The cat is a very intelligent animal, with an acute awareness of the world about it. Usually intelligence is measured as comparison of brain weight with the length of the spinal cord. This shows how much gray matter controls how much body. The cat has a ratio of 4:1 as compared to human's ratio of 50:1.

Learning and Memory

Cats and kittens can learn from their mother or other cats. They can be trained to perform tricks but can't be punished or rewarded like dogs.

A cat uses its learning ability and memory to learn operations like opening a door, tapping on doors, and drinking water from a running faucet, finding its way home and responding to its name by returning home when called.

2. Social Behavior

Cat's communicate in a variety of ways:

- ☆ *Vocalization* – from contented purrs to angry screeches to plaintive mews.
- ☆ *Body signals* – Body postures, facial expressions and tail positions.
- ☆ *Touch* – Rubbing nose, grooming.
- ☆ *Scent* – Tagging territory or identifying individuals.

(a) A Defensive Cat

When faced with a display of aggressive behavior from another animal, a cat's first reaction is to stand its ground. (Cat may have pupils enlarged, ears flattened, mouth open, teeth on show and makes hissing and spitting sounds, fur

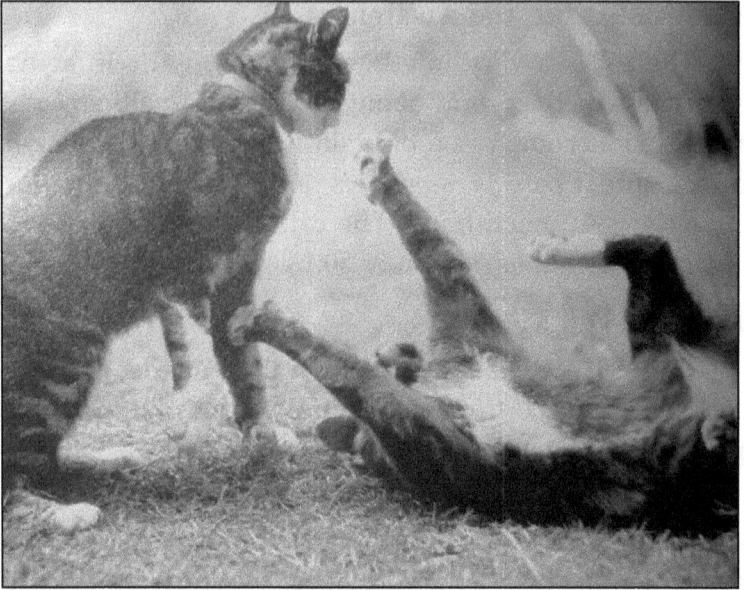

Cat's Playing with Each Other

bristling along back, tail bristling and arched, position arched back and body turned sideways).

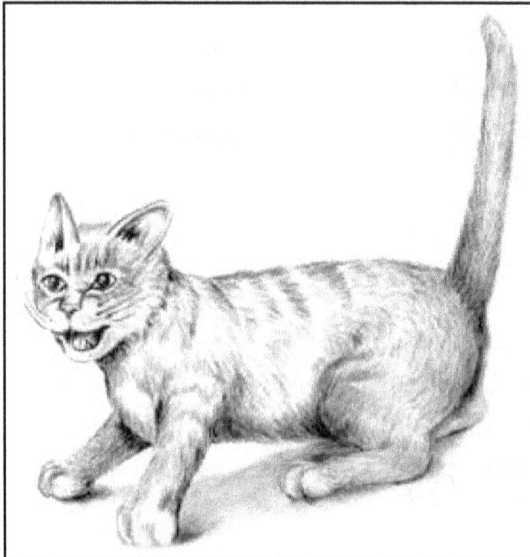

(b) An Aggressive Cat

A dominant cat will use body language to encourage its opponent to turn tail.

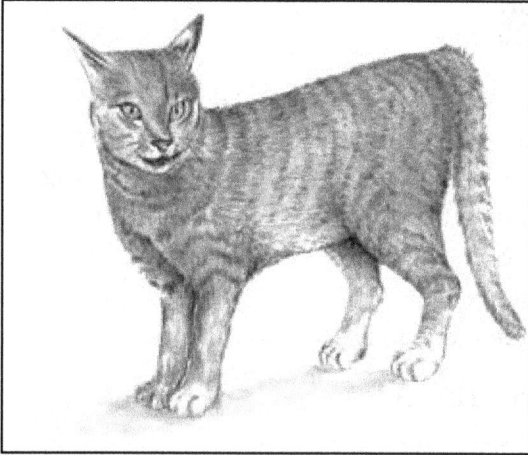

(c) A Submissive Cat

When a cat is faced with an aggressor, it is no match for, it will communicate it's submission by its posture.

Cats are very social animals and they convey personal information by sniffing the other cat's head or beneath its tail as these areas have scent glands.

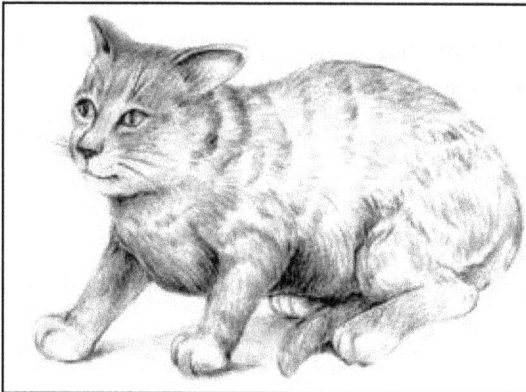

All cats in peck have their positions in the hierarchy. Female cats are organized along matriarchial lines – the unneutered queen with the most kittens is at the top of the pecking order. When a queen is neutered, her social descent is very rapid.

The hierarchical arrangement for male cats is by trial of strength. The roughest, toughest tom becomes the 'top cat' in the area with subordinates of varying ranks and level of authority. This arrangement is rigid, with occasional changes in position, when one member weakens and is overthrown in combat by an ambitious junior. Sometimes a tough outsider can break into the existing local hierarchy.

3. Territorial Areas

Territory is very important to cats, and they stake their claim by marking and defend their area vigorously. Toms control more land than neutered male cats or female cats.

Identification of Cat Territories

It is carried out in three main ways:-

(*a*) Spraying with urine to make "boundary posts"

(*b*) Scratching visual signals on trees or fences with claws

(*c*) Rubbing the head and face against an object to leave the scent from the sebaceous glands.

Anti-social Behavior

Sometimes a lonely or bored cat can behave badly by chewing the carpets, urinating in forbidden spots or biting at its fur. In such cases, you must consult the Vet for advice on remedying the problem.

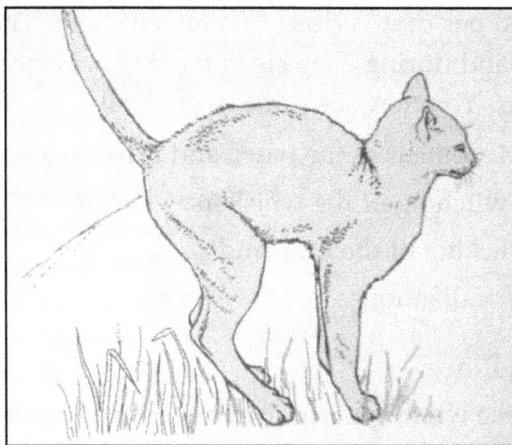

Spraing with Urine

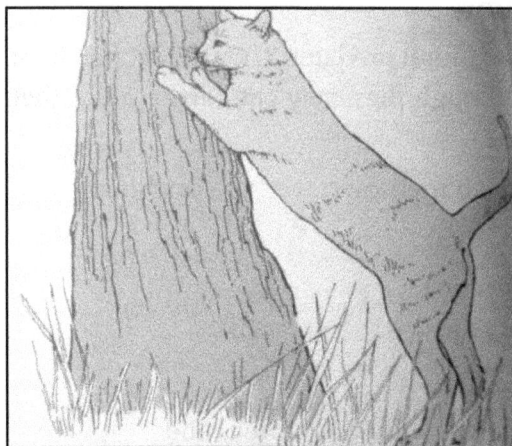

Scratching Tree with Claws

4. Sleep

A cat usually spends a major portion of their life asleep. A cat sleeps on average 16 hours a day, several minutes at a time (the ubiquitous "cat nap"). Awake or asleep cats are constantly receiving and programming information from environment stimuli. Cats have phases of deep and light sleep as 30 per cent is deep, 70 per cent light. The phases alternate, and during deep sleep there is evidence that the cat dreams. You may see some of external signs as:

☆ Movement of the paws and claws,

☆ Twitching of the whiskers,

☆ Flicking of the ears, and

☆ Vocalization.

Sleeping Place

Cats like warm spots to sleep *i.e.,* by the fire, on a sunny windowsill or on a central-heating boiler.

5. Hunting

Cat is a natural predator. They don't often hunt to satisfy hunger, although they may eat part or all of their prey on occasion.

Cats have their own ways of catching:

☆ Stalking,

☆ Pushing,

☆ Ambush,

☆ Attack,

☆ Pinning down the prey, and

☆ The kill.

Chapter 23
Vaccination

Vaccine

Therapeutic material, treated to lose its virulence and containing antigens derived from one or more pathogenic organisms, which on administration to human or other animals, will stimulate active immunity and protect against infection with these or related organisms.

Production of Vaccines

The main principle involved in the production of vaccines is to place virus or bacteria antigens into a liquid. This liquid is introduced in the animal's immune system either by injection or inhalation.

Types of Vaccines

1. Monovalent Vaccines

These vaccines are produced to protect against only one disease *e.g.* Rabies Vaccine.

2. Multivalent Vaccines

These vaccines are prepared to stimulate protection against several diseases at the same time *e.g.* 'Tricat', which is a combination of components to produce protection against feline panleukopenia, calcivirus and rhinotracheitis.

Methods to Prepare the Components

There are three common methods to prepare the vaccines which cause no harm once inoculated into the animal. These are as follows with their advantages and disadvantages:

1. Modified Live Vaccines

In it the live virus particles are altered to an attenuated state. These viruses are in a non-disease causing state but are capable of reproduction and thus will stimulate animal's body to produce antibodies to ward off these virus particles. The immune system responds quickly to vaccination with modified live products than to those which have been killed. The antibodies stimulated by these vaccines are produced in larger quantities and last for a longer period of time.

2. Killed Vaccines

In these vaccines the virus or bacteria is killed in a laboratory and put in a liquid base. These killed particles cannot multiply once inside the animals' body and thus the pet's immune response and antibody production is usually less. So to enhance immune response, killed vaccines usually have more virus or bacterial particles per dose and have added chemicals (adjuvant) and also increase the risk of an allergic reaction to the vaccine.

3. Recombinant Vaccines

In these vaccines, the genes of the virus or bacteria can

be broken and the antigens that produce the best antibody response in an animal can be isolated.

Methods of Administration

There are mainly two methods to administer vaccines:

1. Injectable Vaccines

These are given into the muscle or under the skin. Some vaccines can be given either way; others must only be given one way.

2. Intranasal Vaccines

Some vaccines are manufactured to be given as drops into the nose. These vaccines provide faster protection than those given intramuscularly or subcutaneously. Intranasal vaccines should never be injected into the animal.

Vaccination Schedule of Cat

Age	Vaccination
7 weeks	Combination Vaccine
10 weeks	Combination Vaccine Feline leukemia (FeLV) Chlamydia
12 weeks	Rabies
13 weeks	Combination Vaccine Chlamydia
Adult (boosters)	Combination Vaccine, Chlamydia FeLV Rabies

Adverse Reactions to Vaccination

1. Anaphylaxis

It is a rare, immediate allergic reaction and if untreated, it results in shock, respiratory and cardiac failure and death.

The anaphylactic reaction usually occurs within minutes to hours of the vaccination. Most common symptoms include sudden onset of diarrhea, vomiting, swelling of the face, shock, seizures and death. The heart rate is generally very fast but the pulse is weak. The animal's gums will be very pale and the limbs will feel cold. In such cases your pet need Veterinary attention immediately.

2. Vaccine-Associated Sarcoma

A fibrosarcoma is a tumor of the connective tissue and they tend to invade deeply into the underlying tissues. These tumors are most commonly associated with FeLV vaccine.

A small, painless swelling develops at the site of a recent vaccination. This should disappear in several weeks.

The warning signs for a vaccine-related fibrosarcoma are – a lump persists for more than three months after vaccination, it is still increasing in size even one month after vaccination and it is larger than two centimeters in diameter.

3. Lameness

Lameness can result from several different vaccinations and may last for 3-4 days. Such cases should be treated with fluids, antibiotics and pain medication as per the severity.

4. Swelling at the Injection Site

Some cats may have pain, swelling, redness and irritation at the injection site. If signs persist for more than 1 week, contact your Veterinarian.

5. Birth Defects or Injections

The vaccination of pregnant animals with a modified live vaccine can result in birth defects and in kittens less than 4-5 weeks of age, it can result in developing disease from modified live vaccines.

Effectiveness of Vaccine

Sometimes despite regular and complete vaccinations, the animal may acquire the disease; it is often referred to as 'vaccine failure'. No vaccine can protect every animal to which it is given *i.e.*, even rabies vaccination does not protect every animal from rabies. In most of cases, there is nothing wrong with the vaccine. Rather the wrong is with the body's response to the vaccine.

Some vaccines have short duration of immunity and some have relatively long durations of immunity *i.e.*, some vaccines do not need to be given on an annual basis, but some may need to be given more than once a year.

Causes of 'Vaccine failure'

1. Maternal Antibody

The primary cause of vaccine failure is an interfering level of maternal antibody. These antibodies are transferred from the mother through placenta and colostrums. High levels of maternal antibodies present in a kitten's bloodstream will block the effectiveness of a vaccine. So the age at which kittens can be immunized is proportional to the amount of antibody protection the young animals received from their mother.

2. Insufficient Time Between Vaccination and Exposure

For a vaccine to provide protection, it takes several days to a week or more depending on the animal's body to respond to the vaccine. For some vaccines, an adequate level of immunity usually does not occur until 2-3 weeks after the second vaccination in the series. A young kitten is susceptible to a disease if it is exposed to the disease before a vaccination has had to stimulate the body's immunity. Similarly, a vaccine will not provide protection to a young animal that was already exposed to the disease. The length of protection from a vaccine varies by the disease, type of vaccine, age at vaccination and the immune system of the individual animal.

3. Damage to Vaccine

If not handled properly, a modified live vaccine could be inactivated. If there was a long time period between reconstitution and use or not stored at the proper temperature, then chances of damage to vaccine are more.

4. Inappropriate Administration

Vaccines are developed to be given by a certain route. If a vaccine is administered by a route different from the recommended one, it may not be effective and could cause harm. The entire dose should be given at one time.

5. Vaccination Schedule

The vaccination schedule should be followed properly. If too short of a time elapses between doses of vaccines, there will be vaccine interference. If more than one type of vaccine is to be given, they should be given at the same time and not several days apart.

6. Nutritional Deficiencies

Malnourished animals may not respond to a vaccination properly as deficiency of Vitamin A, Vitamin E and protein deficient diet results in to suppression of the immune system.

Chapter 24
Pet Health Insurance

The owners of the pets are responsible for costs involved in treatment, preventive and emergency care. Insurance companies are coming up with new policies for pets. These pet health insurance policies are similar to human insurance policies and annual premiums depend upon the health of the insured and different coverage plans available.

Insurance companies may look for the following:

☆ What ages of pets are accepted for coverage? The ages may vary depending upon species, breed and life expectancy.

☆ Which breeds are accepted? Who decides what and why is it excluded?

☆ Does policy cover routine examinations, vaccinations and other routine procedures?

☆ What is the amount of coverage in each policy? What is covered and do policy cover certain clinical procedures?

☆ Are pre-existing conditions like diabetes or other genetic ailments are covered or excluded?

☆ Is there any maximum payout?

☆ Are there any reasons for insurance company to cancel the policy?

☆ Are you insured against damage to property if your pet causes injury to other animal or causes an accident?

Chapter 25
Name Tags

Every cat should wear a name tag. Always try to keep your cat's name tag up to date with proper contact number and information. A name tag can be of stainless steel, bras name tags or plates. A name tag can be source of reunion after losing your cat and it can save your family from a painful experience and save your cat's life.

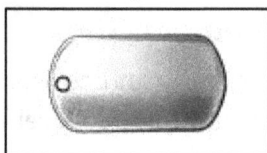

Name Tage for Your Cat

Chapter 26
How to Choose the Right Veterinarian

Choosing a right Veterinarian for you and your cat is not always easy. You must find a Veterinarian with whom you and your pet can feel comfortable and can make a trusting relationship.

Where to Find a Vet

1. Ask friends, family and co-workers about the Vet in your area, comfortable level with Vet and staff, Vet's approach for diagnosis and treatment.

2. *Breed clubs*: You can get the information from a breed club.

3. *Yellow pages*: Yellow pages will provide information on local Vets, addresses and phone numbers.

Things to Look for When Visiting a Vet Clinic

1. Work hours and emergencies:
   - ☆ What are the regular office hours?
   - ☆ How are emergencies handled during work hours, after hours and on holidays?
   - ☆ When doctors are available for appointments?

2. Veterinarian and staff:
   - ☆ Do you feel comfortable with doctor and staff?
   - ☆ How the phone calls are answered and handled?
   - ☆ Are the staff knowledgeable?
   - ☆ Can you see a specific doctor or different doctors?

3. Fees and mode of payment:
   - ☆ What methods of payment are accepted?
   - ☆ Are credit cards accepted?

4. Facilities:
   - ☆ Is the practice neat and clean?
   - ☆ Are the grounds well kept?
   - ☆ Is the facility in a good location and easy for you to get to?

5. Services:
   - ☆ What type of services are available?

     Surgery, Radiology, Dentistry, Ultrasonography, Endoscopy, Laboratory testing, Nutritional counseling, Boarding, Grooming, etc.

Chapter 27
Annual Veterinary Exams

Annual physical exam will review on following aspects:

☆ *Vaccination status*

☆ *Parasite control* – for ectoparasites and endoparasites

☆ *Dental hygiene* – any sign of paleness or gum infection

☆ *Eyes and ears* – any discharge, redness or itching

☆ *Nutrition* – amount of food supplements, water consumption and frequency of feeding

☆ *Breathing* – any coughing, sneezing, nasal discharge

☆ *Coat and skin* – any hair loss, lumps, shedding, mats and itchy spots

☆ *Behavior* – change in temperature, aggression or inappropriate elimination

☆ *Legs* – limping, weakness or toenail problem

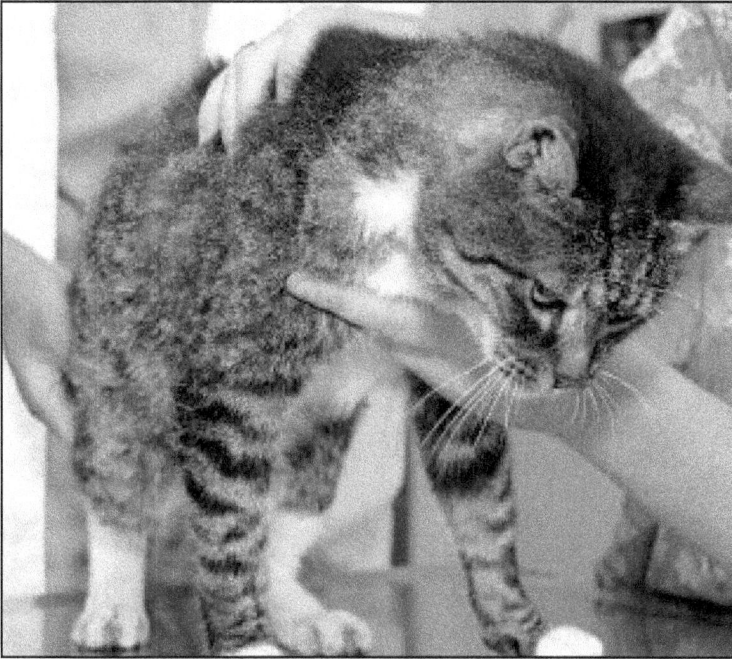

General Examination of Cat

☆ *Digestive system* – any vomiting, diarrhea, constipation, gas or abnormal stools

☆ Blood tests – especially for geriatric cats, with medical problems.

Chapter 28
Care of Older Cats

It is your duty and responsibility to give quality of life to your kitten. You can achieve it through regular checkups and vaccinations. Preventive care can add years and quality to the life of your older cat. You must consider your cat, your Vet and yourself as a team to keep your cat happy and healthy. Regular Veterinary care is essential to keep your cat healthy.

There are various tests which are helpful in diagnosing a problem at very early stage and helpful to start the treatment. Your Veterinarian may recommend various tests and exams as described below:

1. *History*: History is an important tool for your Vet. Monitor your older pet and keeping records of signs of disease will be valuable in making a proper diagnosis.

2. *Physical exam*: Your older cat should receive regular exams and frequency depends upon the health

status of your cat. Make sure to tell your Veterinarian about any conditions you have observed and want to be evaluated by your Vet.

3. *Oral exam*: An oral exam should include an examination of mouth, teeth, gums, throat and tongue.

4. *Ophthalmic exam*: Eyes should be checked on regular basis as any change in the eyes can be an indication of another disease going on in the body or can be due to eye disease itself.

5. *Diet and nutrition*:   Sudden weight gain or weight loss may be the first signs of disease. If your cat weight changes, consult your Vet about it. Your Vet may change the diet plan accordingly.

6. *Parasite control*: The physical exam should include checking for any ectoparasites, if present and your Vet will be able to recommend products to protect your cat from those parasites.

   Likely, a fecal exam should be done routinely to identify internal parasites, if present. Your Vet will recommend which wormer to be used for your cat.

7. *Vaccination*: You must keep your cat up-to-date for his/her vaccinations. Always consult your Vet for vaccine schedule.

8. *Urinalysis*: Urine can be examined to find out any concurrent or underlying disease.

9. *Blood Test*: This may include complete blood count (CBC), liver function test (LFT), kidney function test (KFT), enzymes, hormones, proteins and electrolytes etc.

10. *Radiography*: Radiographs (X-rays) may be helpful to find out any complication, if present. Otherwise, normal radiograph will give a baseline for further evaluation.

11. *Blood pressure*: This can be used as one of the diagnostic tool.

Behavior Changes in Older Cats

As the cats become older, they are more likely to develop few behavioral problems. Out of these some can be corrected, if diagnosed and treated appropriately.

1. Aggression

A cat may become aggressive due to different reasons like pain (arthritis), vision or hearing loss or any type of stress. If your cat is becoming aggressive, consult your Vet to help cat.

2. Inappropriate Elimination

In most of the older cats urinating or defecating outside the litter box is one of the common behavior problems. Such cat should be properly examined by your Vet for any medical problem *i.e.*, diabetes, hyperthyroidism, any liver or kidney disease, arthritis, loss of vision or anal sac disease. In cats stress can be a major factor for improper elimination. Stress can be due to change of place, change in routine or change in family structure. To reduce this factor you must keep your cat in a quiet portion of the house during packing and while shifting always keep your cat in a quiet corner of your new home as well. Make it comfortable by placing her food, water, liter box in that room and try to spend some quality time. Always feed her and clean the litter box at the usual time. Now gradually let her become familiar to the rest of the house.

Other way to control this behavior is to feed the cat in areas in which she is inappropriately eliminating and use pet repellents to limit her access to these areas.

3. Anxiety

Some cats show fear or anxiety. You must find out the cause of anxiety for its control and treatment.

The Ageing Process

The older cats definitely show signs of aging. We can help them by diagnosing the problems at early stage and by treating them properly and providing them suitable environment.

1. Nutritional Needs

Obesity is not a common problem in older cats, rather they tend to lose some fat. So, older cats require easily digestible fat to get the same amount of energy. You need to monitor the condition and body weight of your cat and adjust the diet accordingly.

2. Hair Coat

Older cats may show gray hair and may become thinner and duller but this can also be a sign of nutritional deficiency. Usually cats groom themselves very well but older cats may need to be groomed often. During grooming session you can check for lumps, sores or any bumps and can give attention to anal area.

3. Nails

In older cats, nails may tend to become brittle. Such nails must be trimmed carefully and you may need to clip them more often as your cat may not use scratch post often.

4. Decreased Mobility

Older cats may develop arthritis and may have difficulty in jumping or walking over the stairs. These cats need regular exercise as a part of their routine to keep their systems well. You may need to provide low-sided litter boxes and cat beds to these cats. Make sure the litter box and food and water bowls are at the same level of the house where the cat spends most of her time.

5. Constipation

This is very common problem in older cats and very painful for cats with arthritis or anal gland disease. Cats that drink less water have more tendencies to develop constipation. This could be a sign of other diseases and should be evaluated by your Veterinarian.

6. Dental Diseases

The teeth should be checked and cleaned regularly. Any dental disease may develop life-threatening complications, so it may need regular checkups and professional cleaning.

7. Hearing Loss

Older cats usually have hearing loss. Slight hearing loss is hard to evaluate and often it is very severe before the owner becomes aware of the problem. Aggression could be the first sign of this problem. This effect cannot be reversed, but some changes in interaction can reduce the effects. These cats can sense vibrations, so even clapping hands may alert the cat to your presence.

8. Vision Loss

Your cat may experience vision loss as they grow older. Any sudden changes in vision may be an alarm for you to take the cat to Vet for ophthalmic exam.

9. Immune System

The older cat is more prone to develop infection as their immune system does not work very well. So it is important to keep your cat's vaccination up to date.

10. Heart and Lung Functions

Cats can develop heart problems as they grow older. They are more prone to have a disease of heart muscle called cardiomyopathy. Diagnostic tests like radiograph (X-rays) and an ECG can be helpful in diagnosing the heart disease.

Similarly, lungs also lose their elasticity and the ability of the lungs to oxygenate the blood may be decreased and can develop respiratory infections.

11. Liver Function

Liver has the ability to detoxify the blood and produce various enzymes and proteins. This functioning is reduced as the cat ages. Sometimes normal cat may show elevated levels or sick animals may show normal levels of liver enzymes. This makes interpretation of these tests very difficult. Before anesthetic procedures it is always good to check for the blood tests values to adjust the dose of drugs, if required.

13. Mammary Glands

Older female cats should have mammary glands checked as part of the regular physical exam. Unsprayed female cats may have more tendencies to develop mammary tumor and unfortunately approximately 85 per cent of these tumors in cats are malignant.

14. Behavior Changes

Older cats may have behavior changes *i.e.* aggression, increased vocalization, inappropriate elimination and noise phobia. Stress may be a major factor for all these, so you need to reduce the stress to make her comfortable.

Some Signs of Common Diseases

Signs	Associated Diseases
☆ Weight gain	☆ Obesity
☆ Weight loss	☆ Kidney diseases
	☆ Liver diseases
	☆ Gastrointestinal diseases
	☆ Hyperthyroidism
	☆ Hepatic lipidosis
	☆ IBD
	☆ Dental diseases
☆ Behavior changes	☆ Liver diseases
	☆ Kidney diseases
	☆ Vision or hearing loss
	☆ Pain
☆ Change in activity level	☆ Pain
	☆ Obesity
	☆ Anemia
	☆ Arthritis
	☆ Diabetes
	☆ Hyperthyroidism
☆ Coughing	☆ Asthma
	☆ Cancer
	☆ Respiratory diseases
☆ Vomiting	☆ Kidney diseases
	☆ Liver diseases
	☆ GI diseases
	☆ IBD

Contd...

Signs	Associated Diseases
☆ Diarrhea	☆ GI diseases
	☆ IBD
	☆ Liver diseases
	☆ Kidney diseases
☆ Bad breath	☆ Dental diseases
	☆ Kidney diseases
☆ Seizures	☆ Liver diseases
	☆ Kidney diseases
	☆ Cancer
	☆ Epilepsy
☆ Lameness	☆ Arthritis
	☆ Obesity
☆ Urinary incontinence	☆ Pain
	☆ IBD
	☆ Cancer
	☆ Bladder stones
	☆ Kidney diseases

Contact your Vet when your cat shows these signs.

The following briefing will help you to decide between the emergency conditions or 'wait and watch' conditions.

Emergency Conditions

Contact your Vet immediately if your cat –

1. Shows Your Signs of Heart or Respiratory Disease

☆ No pulse or heart beat

☆ No breathing or dyspnea

☆ Bluish or white gum

2. **Had Trauma like**

    ☆ A broken bone

    ☆ An eye injury or head trauma

    ☆ Heavy bleeding

    ☆ A scorpion bite or snake bite

    ☆ A fight with another animal

    ☆ Accidentally hit by a vehicle

    ☆ A wound from a bullet or punctured wounds to the abdomen

    ☆ A severe lacerated wound or a gaping wound

    ☆ Falling or jumping from an open window, balcony or roof

3.. **Had Heat or Cold Related Injuries**

    ☆ Burns or inhaled smoke

    ☆ Heat stroke or hyperthermia or fever

    ☆ Hypothermia or frostbite

4. **Has Signs of Gastrointestinal Disease Including**

    ☆ Vomiting

    ☆ Diarrhea with blood and foul smell

    ☆ Black, tarry stool

    ☆ Constipation

    ☆ Choking

    ☆ Rectal prolapse

5. **Has Signs of Urinary or Reproductive Problems**

    ☆ Blood from the urinary or genital tracts

    ☆ Sowing signs of pain while trying to urinate

☆ Straining continuously, but unable to pass urine

☆ Difficulty in giving birth *i.e.*, no kitten after 24 hrs. of beginning labor, Abnormal bleeding, infrequent contractions once labor has started

6. **Shows Symptoms of Muscular or Nervous Diseases**

☆ Seizures

☆ Lethargy, unconsciousness or coma

☆ Severe pain

☆ Sudden inability to bear weight on one or more limbs.

If your cat shows following signs take your cat the same day to your Vet:

1. **Signs of Heart or Respiratory Diseases**

☆ Continuous sneezing or coughing

☆ Difficulty breathing

2. **Signs Related to Gastrointestinal Diseases**

☆ Vomiting or diarrhea for more than 24 hrs.

☆ Not eating or drinking for more than 24 hrs.

☆ Drinking water excessively

3. **Signs Related to Urinary or Reproductive Problems**

☆ A male dog with swollen testicles or scrotum

☆ A retained after birth for over 8 hrs.

4. **Signs of Nervous or Muscular Disease Including**

☆ Sudden change in behavior

☆ Sudden, severe lameness

☆ Crying when touched

☆ Cloudy eyes

5. **Signs Associated with Skin Diseases**

☆ A rash, continuous scratching, excessive head shaking

☆ Maggots

☆ Abnormal lumps, which are red and painful.

Contact your Vet in 24 hrs. If your cat shows signs related to:

1. **Digestive System**

☆ Not eating, but no other ailment

☆ Foul breath

☆ Drooling

☆ Occasional vomiting

☆ A soft stool without any blood, mucus or pain

2. **Nervous System**

☆ Swollen joints

☆ Lethargy, depression

☆ Lameness for more than 24 hours

3. **Skin**

☆ Moderate itching

☆ A discharge from the eye or ear.

Chapter 29
Breeding

Female cats reach sexual maturity between 7-12 months and males between 10-14 months.

The Queen's Cycle

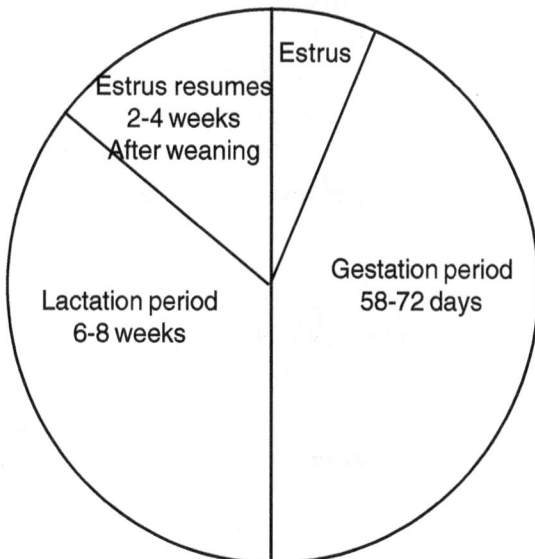

Estrus

Estrus resumes
2-4 weeks
After weaning

Gestation period
58-72 days

Lactation period
6-8 weeks

Pregnancy

If the mating has been successful, your queen won't come back into estrus and will soon show signs of pregnancy. However, if she hasn't conceived, estrus will recur two to three weeks later. The gestation length is about nine weeks.

Signs of Pregnancy

☆ Gradual weight gain – 2 – 4 lbs, depending on the number of kittens

☆ Reddening nipples – it is known as "pinking-up", and occurs about the third week of   pregnancy.

☆ Swollen abdomen – don't palpate the abdomen too hard, as you could cause serious damage.

☆ Behavior changes – becomes maternal

Preparation of a Kittening Box

When the queen is within two weeks of giving birth, try to keep her indoors and prepare a kittening box. The box should be put in a warm, comfortable and isolated place and lined with lots of newspaper (a good insulator, clean and easy to change). Once the box is ready, introduce the queen to it. If she selects an alternative site, move the box there.

The Birth

When the time to give birth arrives, some hormones in queen's body begin the process of ejecting the kittens from the uterus. Average length of a cat's pregnancy is 65 days, birth may commence anytime from one week before to one week after this date.

Stages of Labor

1. First Stage

This stage may last up to six hours and begins when the cervix opens up and a "wedge" of fetal membranes from the uterus enters it. As this happens, the involuntary contractions of the uterine muscles begin the new kitten's journey to the outside world. When the contractions begin, the queen will probably go to her kittening bed. She may start breathing more rapidly, panting and purring, but not in distress. A clear vaginal discharge may be seen and at the end of the first stage clear or slightly cloudy water or a little blood is released.

2. Second Stage

This stage should last for 10-30 minutes and no longer than 90 minutes. It starts when the emerging fetus and its membranes stimulate the mother to aid the involuntary uterine contractions with voluntary abdominal muscle contractions or straining. The queen starts licking at her vulva and won't move from her kittening box. Soon, a cloudy gray bleb appears at the vulval opening. The interval between bouts of bearing down decreases, until straining occurs once every 15-30 seconds. With a number of final contractions the queen pushes out the kitten.

3. Third Stage

Once the kitten has emerged, the expulsion of the membranes and placenta usually follows very quickly. The birth of each kitten is a separate labor, with its own three stages. Each kitten has its own membranes and placenta, except in case of identical twins, where they may share one set.

Helping an Inexperienced Queen

Sometimes a first-time mother won't lick the kitten, break open the membranes where necessary, or sever the umbilical cord. In such a case, you will have to intervene immediately or the kitten may die.

1. If the membranes are still covering the new-born kitten, simply rip them off.

2. Next, rub the kitten with dry towel, clear the nostrils for any type of mucus blockage.

3. Once the kitten is breathing and wriggling, you can attend to the umbilical cord. Begin by immersing some strong cotton and a pair of scissors in antiseptic. Tie the cotton tightly around the umbilical cord about 1 inch from the navel.

4. Knot the cotton and then cut the cord 3/16 inch beyond the cotton on the placental side of the knot.

5. Finally, place the kitten in a box.

After the Birth of a Kitten

As soon as a kitten is born, the queen starts licking it and she bites off the umbilical cord 1–1.5 inches from its navel. She may try to eat the placenta – this behavior is instinctive in many mammals *i.e.,* to remove any material that might attract scavenging. Try to remove it before she eats it as it may give her indigestion. But if she does eat it, don't worry – it won't harm her.

Helping a Weak Kitten

If a kitten is very cold and feeble at birth, immerse it up to its neck in a bowl of water (101°F). Keep hold of the kitten by the head and stroke and massage its body gently under the water. After 2-3 minutes it should become more vigorous. Take it out of the water and dry it carefully with warm toweling. Place it in a warm box.

Total Kittening Length

The time between the births of successive kitten can vary from 5 minutes to two hours. Sometimes a queen will deliver half a litter, and then suspend operations for 12-24 hours before delivering the rest. If this happens, you may be worried. If the first group of kittens were delivered normally and at short intervals and the queen appears content and accepts food, there may be no need to worry. A delay can be confused with "uterine inertia", and the queen tires of bearing down, eventually giving up. This condition is not normal, and needs Veterinarian attention. An affected queen usually appears more fatigued and disinterested than a resting cat, but the difference can be difficult to judge. Thus, if your cat has not finished giving birth and two hours have elapsed since the last kitten was born, call the Vet.

Post Natal Check List

☆ Change the bedding as soon as kittening is over.

☆ Give a quality and well balanced diet.

☆ Keep queen indoors for 3-4 days, but keep the kittens inside until weaned.

Labor Problems

1. Difficult Labor

A kitten can jam in the birth canal. It may be a wrong presentation or the kitten may be abnormally large. If a kitten is partly out of the vulva and the queen is having difficulty getting it any further; wash your hands, then lubricate the kitten and vulval entrance with petroleum jelly or soap flakes in a little warm water. Firmly, but gently grasp the kitten and try to ease it out. Do not jerk or pull hard on the kitten, though twisting it slightly may help you to pull it out.

2.   Caesarian Section

It is quick, low-risk and does not interfere with the mother's ability to rear her young or have subsequent litters.

3.   An Off-color Queen

Queen will need to rest after long labor and may seem quite weak for a while. But by the following day she should start settling down to rearing her kittens and resume normal eating and drinking. If this is not the case, you must contact the Vet immediately.

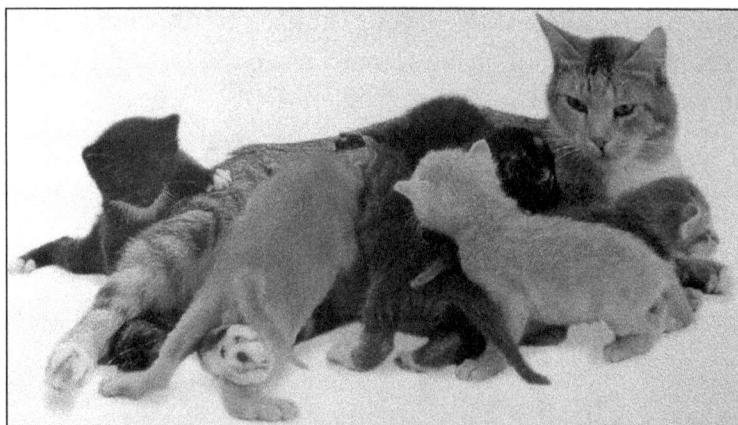

Care of Queen and Newborn

Feeding

The queen should be allowed to access food, water and a litter box within 2-3 days, the queen's appetite will double from her pre-pregnancy intake. She will need a constant supply of a high quality kitten food and water to maintain her weight and health while feeding the kittens. She should weigh the same at weaning as she did when she was bred.

Kittens nurse about every 1-2 hours. If their stomach appears round and they sleep quietly, they are eating enough. If they are crying and moving a lot, they are not eating enough. Weak kittens will lay still and not cry. Kittens develop a preference for which teat they nurse from within days of birth. They locate the same teat by smell. Usually, the queen will lick the stomach and perianal area before, during and after nursing to stimulate urination and defecation. She will continue to do this for 2-3 weeks.

A normal kitten weighs 100 g + 10 g at time of birth. The kittens less than 90 g at birth are likely to die within the first days of life. They may lose weight in first 24 hours after birth but minimal weight gain should be 7-10 g daily and it should be double the birth weight within the first 14 days of life. Failure of weight gain is first sign of illness in kittens.

Initially kitten food can be mixed with milk replacer and hot water and should be given at least 3-4 meals a day. Gradually every week decrease the amount of the milk replacer and water and increase the quantity of dry food. By the age of 7-8 weeks, the kittens are eating dry food and should be weaned completely from mother's milk and should use the litter box.

During weaning process, the amount of food for dam should be decreased gradually. During the fifth week of lactation, queen's diet should be changed to adult food and slowly decrease the amount of kitten food. By the eighth week of lactation, the queen should be on adult food.

Mother's Health

Queen's mammary glands and nipples should be checked for any redness, hardness or discharge. If there is any infection in the mammary glands, the veterinarian should be consulted immediately to prevent its spread. The kitten's nails should be trimmed regularly and deciduous teeth start coming in around day 11, so the mammary glands should be checked daily for bites or scratches.

Initially, the Queen has a heavy bloody discharge from her vulva for several days. It decreases in amount, become darker and almost gone within 2-3 weeks.

Kitten Health Development

Kittens should be examined by the veterinarian as soon as possible after birth for cleft palate. A complete health check up should be done by a Veterinarian at 6-7 weeks of age for hernias, parasites, eye diseases and ear mites.

The infections of the umbilicus are rare and the umbilical cord normally falls off in 2-3 days. Kittens twitch and jerk

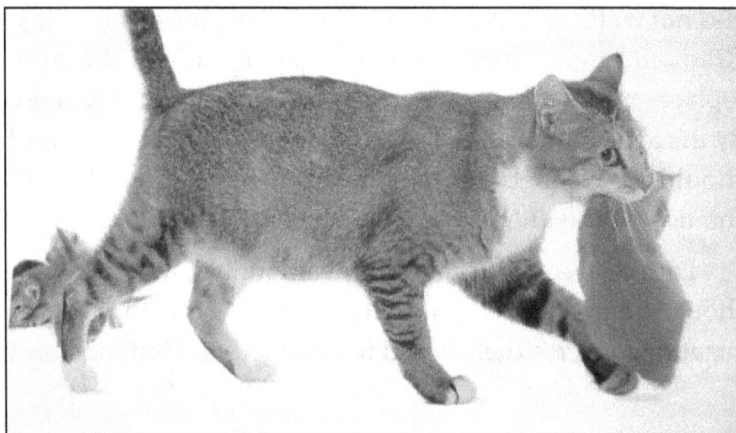

during sleeping as it helps in development of muscular and nervous systems.

The kitten's eyes will open around 7-10 days of age. Some kittens will take a day to open the eyes while the others may take 3-4 days. Do not try to open the lids as the immature retina is not ready to handle light. If the eyes have white or deep blue color, you must take it to the vet immediately.

The ears open around two weeks of age and they should hear clearly by 4 weeks of age. Usually white cats with blue eyes are deaf and the gene causing deafness is associated to gene responsible for producing coat and eye color combination.

The milk teeth start to erupt at 2-4 weeks of age and all deciduous teeth are present by 8 weeks of age.

A good scratch post should be available to kittens by 3 weeks of age. They learn to use scratch post by imitating the mother and once learnt will be followed for whole life.

Hygiene and litter box – the nesting box should be changed every day. At about four weeks of age, the kittens begin moving, scratching and play in it. Slowly, by six weeks of age, they learn to eliminate in the litter box and learn to bury their faces by watching the Queen burying hers.

Temperature – the temperature should be maintained at about 75-80°F for the first week and can be dropped to about 70°F gradually. Kittens usually lay side by side or on the top of each other to stay warm. If they are spread throughout the box, the temperature may be too warm. Initially, the kittens are unable to regulate their body temperature and need the extra heat.

How to Raise Orphans

The mother Queen who either cannot produce enough milk or has behavioral or psychological abnormalities, *i.e.,* lacks maternal instincts may abandon the kittens. In some rare cases, the mother may be dead or may be sick and not able to take care of the kittens. For successful rearing of these kittens, it is necessary to follow a regular schedule of feedings, playing, sleeping in a healthy and safe environment. It is difficult but possible to raise one orphaned kitten or an entire litter. For the successful rate one must consider the following points:

1. Nutrition

If the mother allow the kittens to nurse, your work load will be reduced otherwise you need to bottle or tube fed the kitten. Bottle feeding is recommended over tube feeding and kitten should be fed while he is on his belly and not on his back. Readymade kitten milk formulas and homemade milk formula are also available. Commercial preparations are readily available and are nutritionally balanced while homemade recipes are not perfectly balanced but can meet the demand for few days.

Homemade Preparation

Condensed milk + water + yoghurt + 4 small egg yolks

Do not use cow's milk or goat's milk for as milk replacer. Do not give egg white as it may lead to biotin deficiency.

Whether using a commercial or homemade formula, make formula for one day and keep it in the refrigerator. Warm the milk replacer till 98-100°F before feeding and mix well before use. Always wash and dry the bottles and nipples between feedings.

Bottle feeding needs to be done carefully to prevent aspiration pneumonia. So the kittens need to be burped during and after each feeding. Hold them over your shoulder and pat their back.

The first 24-48 hours each kitten needs 1 ml of milk per hour. Gradually each day increase the amount per meal by 0.5 ml until a maximum of 10 ml/meal is reached and kittens will need 9 – 12 feedings per day.

Orphan Kitten Feeding Schedule

Weeks Postpartum	Feedings per Day	Volume of Formula per Meal (ml)	Body Weight (grams)
1	9–12	1–8	100–200
2	9	8–10	200–300
3	8	10	300–350
4	7	10	350–400
5	6	8	400–500
6	5	Solid food intro...	450–600
7	4	–do–	500–750

2. Sanitation

A newborn kitten is unable to urinate or defecate as he lacks the necessary muscle control over these functions. In normal cases, the mother licks the kitten's anal area to stimulate urination and defecation. So, orphaned kittens must be manually stimulated after each and every feeding by the owner to enable urination and defecation. Some kittens will respond better before eating while others respond better after eating. Most kittens will eliminate on their own by three weeks of age.

Observe the urine and faeces for signs of ill health. The urine should be a pale yellow or clear. Do not feed more formula at one time, but feed more often. Green colored stool indicates infection and too hard stool indicates not enough formula. Excess feeding causes gas, bloating, regurgitation and aspiration into the lungs.

3.   Temperature

Always keep a room thermometer under the light source to monitor the temperature. For the first week, air temperature should be maintained at 85-90°F and a relative humidity of 55-65 per cent. Over the next 3 weeks, decrease the temperature to 75°F. If the kittens are piled on top of each other all the time, they are cold. By about 4 weeks of age, the kittens' body temperature is in the range of 100–102°F. Always try to use blanket or newspapers as bed for the kittens, as it will help in the development of their motor functions.

4.   Socialization

Orphaned kittens need more mental and physical stimulation as compared to other kittens. They need to be petted and cuddled quite often and it is necessary for such kittens to have interaction with human beings by the age of 3-5 weeks. If they have other littermates, they will stimulate each other while moving. Early socialization is a useful tool for the kittens to feel secure and to avoid future behavior problems.

Chapter 30
Spaying

Ovario-hysterectomy (spaying) is the best way and ideal approach to reduce the number of unwanted kittens. Some people believe that motherhood will help Queen to become a better, calm and affectionate pet or to mature completely. These believe are not true. Pregnancy and motherhood do not help in physical or mental development of cat and maturity level of the Queen remains unaltered. It is very difficult to find good homes for all the kittens and in some cases all pregnancies don't go smoothly. There could be problems like difficult labor, kitten death and other potential health problems like uterus infection and mammary gland complications.

Most of the clients usually end up with the decision that they had never wished a litter from their Queen. Finally, if you don't want kittens, then ask your vet for the spaying of your female cat. To leave her unmated and unoperated is not the solution as they have tendency to develop ovarian cyst and other uterine conditions when they grow older. Spaying (ovario-hysterectomy) involves the removal of ovaries, oviducts, uterine horns and body of uterus. It is irreversible in nature and has no after effects.

This surgical procedure not only prevents the pregnancy but also eliminates the heat cycles, as the surgery removes the source of production of hormones responsible for heat cycles.

Disadvantages of Now Spaying Your Cat

1. *Estrus or heat period* – Cats ovulate, only if she get mated. If not mated in the heat period, she will come back in to heat every 2 to 3 weeks until mating happens. These cats often develop behavior problems, *i.e.*, try to escape from home or may start howling at any time. Some unspayed females may spray urine when they are in heat.

2. *Pyometra* – Unspayed cats may develop uterine infection, *i.e.*, uterine horns becomes filled with pus. This condition is fatal, if left untreated and only treatment for this is ovario-hysterectomy.

3. *Tumors* – Cats may develop uterine and ovarian tumors and spaying is the only option to avoid this condition.

4. *Mammary Cancer* – Cats may develop mammary cancer because of reproductive hormones. Spaying reduces this incidence by 40-60 per cent.

Important Factors which Prevent Spaying

1. Do not spay a kitten less than 3 months old.

2. Do not spay a cat during estrus as there will be more bleeding.

3. No Queen more than 4 weeks pregnant should be spayed.

4. Spaying a lactating Queen should be avoided and they should be usually spayed at least 2 weeks after the kittens are weaned.

Neutering

Unless you have a breeding stud, all toms should be castrated. This will control behavioral and medical problems. Vasectomies are not preferred in veterinary medicine because all undesired characteristics are caused by the hormone – testosterone, which is produced within the testicle.

Advantages of Neutering

1. Behavioral Advantages

(a) *Reduced fighting* – Castration controls the aggression in cats and thus reduces fighting incidences.

(b) *Decreased spraying* – Urine spraying is a normal but unwanted phenomenon in toms. Neutering is helpful in controlling this habit.

(c) *Straying* – Neutering helps in controlling the roaming of tom cats especially when any female is in heat.

2. Medical Advantages

(a) *Reduced injuries* – Neutering avoids involvement of tom cats in serious fights and thus they don't develop bite wound and abscesses like unneutered tom cats.

(b) *Prevent unplanned litters* – Neutering will also help in preventing unplanned litters.

(c) *Improved Genetics* – Best animals can be selected and kept for breeding, while other toms can be neutered to control unwanted hereditary traits.

Age for Neutering

Male cats can be neutered at 5-6 months of age. Some shelters and Veterinarians neuter them at a younger age, *i.e.*, 8-14 weeks of age. Early neutering does not produce any side effects on growth, physical and behavioral development. Most important point to be considered is safe anesthetics and procedure can be modified accordingly. It is also a fact that animals neutered at a younger age recover faster from anesthesia than the older animals.

Chapter 31
Some Myths

Fatty and Laziness

It is not true that spaying or neutering make them fat and lazy. The main problem is not surgery, it is owner. Neutering and spaying changes the metabolism of cat and they do not need same amount of food. This overfeeding is the main cause that they put on more weight. Secondly, they do not get proper amount of exercise and their activity level also depends on owner's choice. Usually they don't get opportunity for play and exercise and they become fat and lazy.

Spaying after One Heat

Veterinarians do not recommend that one heat is necessary before spaying. Firstly, even first heat can bring the chance of pregnancy and it could affect your cat's health. Secondly, your cat may meet with an accident as they usually run away from home or try to escape from home.

Thirdly, the cats in heat may spray urine and howl at any point of time. Last but not the least; heat may increase the incidence of occurrence of mammary tumors.

Chapter 32

Health Care

A healthy cat 's eyes are clear and bright, nostrils are clean and dry, fur is sleek and unbroken, appetite is good and excretory system functions regularly. It grooms itself regularly and produces no signs of pain or discomfort. The first signs of ill-health usually involve behavior *i.e.*, cat becomes duller, less active and introverted. Its appetite is often affected – may decrease or increase.

Signs of Illness

Acute Signs

If your cat displays any of the following signs consult a Vet immediately – collapse, frequent vomiting for more than 24 hrs, frequent diarrhea for more than 24 hrs, troubled breathing, bleeding from an orifice or dilated pupils.

Major Signs

Vomiting, diarrhea, abnormal breathing, bleeding, scratching, and looking off-color.

Other Common Signs

☆ *Respiratory signs* – sneezing, nasal discharge, coughing.

☆ Oral signs – drooling, over/under eating, increased thirst.

☆ *Eye signs* – discharge, cloudiness.

☆ *Ear signs* – pain when touched, limping.

☆ *Urinary signs* – constipation, urination, straining.

How to Take a Cat's Temperature

The normal temperature of a cat is about 101°F to 102.2°F.

Method

Ask a helper to hold the cat firmly. Use a clinical thermometer; lubricate the glass bulb with mineral oil and insert the thermometer into the anus, until about 1 m of it is inside the cat. Gently angle the thermometer so that the

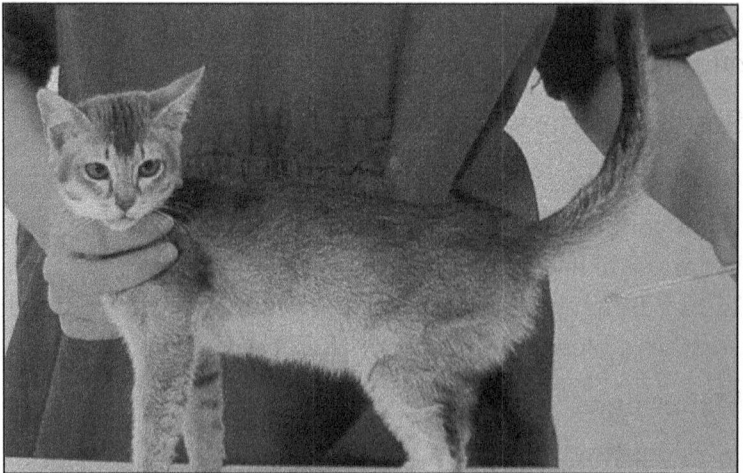

Checking the Cat's Temperature

bulb comes into contact with the wall of the rectum. Hold it in position for about one minute, then withdraw, wipe and read it against the scale.

Common Systematic Disorders

Respiratory Disorders

Pneumonia

Main clinical signs are labored, rapid breathing, loss of appetite and malaise. Causative agents are bacterial or fungal infection, inhalation of liquids, and irritation by gases or parasites.

Bronchitis

This condition is indicated by a cough, and is caused by inflammation of the air tubes. Main causes include gas, smoke, foreign bodies or infections.

Pleurisy

It is a condition in which chest cavity is filled with milky, purulent fluid that compresses the lung and makes breathing difficult. In most of cases the unknown causative factor.

Asthma

Asthmatic attacks are characterized by heavy, distressed breathing and wheezing. In most of the cases, the major cause is allergic sensitivity.

Cat Flu

Main clinical symptoms include inflammation of the eye, nose, and windpipe with resultant discharge. The cat becomes feverish, loses its appetite and sneezes continually. In complicated cases the eyes and nostrils become thicker and purulent. Prevention is better than treatment and can be achieved by proper and regular vaccination of your cat.

Digestive Disorders

Tooth Decay

The cat's which are on minced or canned food, have a tendency to accumulate tartar or scale around their teeth. The tartar leads to gingivitis (inflammation of gums) and slowly the infection creeps down the socket to cause periodontal disease. As a result of it, the tooth may become loose and extraction will be necessary. To prevent such condition, a cat's teeth must be kept clean.

Gastritis

It is inflammation of stomach and is usually caused by either the ingestion of poisons or irritant chemicals. The cat may vomit, feel thirsty and may have malaise. If these symptoms are severe, contact your Vet immediately.

Hairball

Cats who groom themselves very frequently are prone to swallow hairs, which gradually build up into a soggy, dark-colored mass in the stomach. If the hairball is not regurgitated or passed through the intestine, the cat may lose weight gradually.

Obesity

Persistent overfeeding could result in to obesity, which may put strain on the heart, liver and joints.

Diarrhea

In some cats, chronic diarrhea may be due to deficiency of the enzyme lactase or to an allergy to milk protein. In such cases, milk should be excluded from the diet. In severe cases of diarrhea, Vet should be consulted immediately.

Constipation

Older cats are more prone to develop impaction of the large intestine and rectum. Cat may strain hard to pass the stool, show signs of pain, have crouchy posture and gradually become dull. For treatment, consult your Vet.

Eye Problems

Scratched Eyelid or Eye

The most common cause is a scratch from another cat. Affected cat will show soreness, watering, blinking, swollen eyelids and purulent discharge.

Conjunctivitis

It is inflammation of the lining of the eyelids and the thin layer of tissue covering the visible white of the eyeball. Signs include redness, watering, soreness, blinking and closure of the lids. Conjunctivitis can be caused by bacterial and viral infections, allergic reaction, a foreign body or irritant gases.

Corneal Problems

The normal transparent 'window' of the eye may be damaged by bacteria or by becoming cloudy and bluish, and later white and opaque. Simple, non-infected corneal wounds heal quickly, but where infections are present, ulceration or further inflammation deeper in the eye may follow.

Glaucoma

This condition involves enlargement of the eye with corneal cloudiness, and occurs when the fluid within the eye can't circulate as a result of internal bleeding, inflammation of the iris or a tumor.

Cataracts

Opacity of the pupil of a cat's eye is generally due to the development of a cataract in the lens. Another reason may be a change in the refractive index of the lens due to age.

Cherry Eye

The third eyelid or nictating membrane due to damage and inflammation protrudes at the corner of the eye.

Ear Problems

Canker

The outer ear inflammation is caused by the presence of foreign bodies such as bacteria, fungi, or mites. An affected cat will scratch its ears, shake its head, show signs of irritation and sometimes discharge as well. Mange mites are the most common cause, resulting in irritation of the ear canal and secretion of a wax.

Puffy Ear

Cats which scratch violently at their ears often burst blood vessels in the ear flap. This will produce hematoma and cat will carry on scratching due to irritation and may tilt its head to the affected side.

Urinary Tract Disorders

Acute Renal Failure

Most common signs are vomiting, thirst, severe dullness, convulsions and coma.

Chronic Renal Failure

Sings include great thirst, increased urinary output, weight loss, uremia, vomiting, bad breath, dehydration and ulcerated mouth.

Urinary Incontinence

If your cat urinates elsewhere, the possible cause could be territorial marking, diabetes, bladder inflammation or damage to the bladder.

Straining

Your cat may strain because of constipation, intestinal blockage, cystitis, urinary stones or onset of labor.

Reproductive Disorders

Pyometra

It mean pus in the uterus. Signs may include vulval discharge, dullness, increased thirst, loss of appetite, vomiting, enlargement of the abdomen and poor body condition.

Ovarian Cysts

When ovarian follicles don't ripen, instead enlarge into cysts and turn out large quantities of female sex hormone. Signs include infertility, permanent heat periods, loss of weight, and a generally discontented temperament.

Metritis

Infection of the uterus and inflammation may follow a difficult birth. Signs may include dullness, lack of appetite, fever, pain in the abdomen, smelly vulval discharge, exercise thirst and vomiting.

Mammary Gland Problems

Signs may include swelling, redness, dullness, tenderness, disinterest in food and refusing to let the kitten suckle.

Lactation Tetany

It is also called as eclampsia or milk fever and is caused by a low calcium level in the blood. Signs may include muscular twitching, tremors, spasm, paralysis, panting and vomiting.

Circulatory Disorders

Heart Disease

As cats get older, the heart valve may get weaker or become blocked. Signs include heavy breathing or breathlessness, a tendency to tire easily, coughing, wheezing, gasping and respiratory distress, liver enlargement, intestinal upsets and nervous signs.

Anemia

It is a reduction in number of circulating red blood cells or the amount of oxygen carrying hemoglobin within those cells is known as anemia. Three main reasons for this are:

1. The destruction of red blood cells by parasites, bacterial toxin.
2. Loss of blood due to an accident, a bleeding ulcer or the presence of blood-sucking parasites.
3. Reduced or abnormal production of new R.B.C.s in the bone marrow as a result of a tumor, an acute infection, a chronic septic condition, chronic kidney disease etc.

Leukemia

It is a cancerous multiplication of white blood cells caused by a virus. It is contagious and spread by direct contact. Signs may include anemia, weakness, and loss of weight, vomiting, diarrhea and respiratory problems.

Neurological Problems

Meningitis

The membranes covering of the brain and spinal cord become inflamed, and it is usually caused by the spread of infection from other parts of the body. Signs include dullness, depression, and fever, loss of appetite, convulsions and dilated pupils.

Encephalitis

It is inflammation of the brain itself and can be caused by bacteremia, septicemia, and bacteria spreading from an infected middle or inner ear, virus, fungi and protozoan. Signs will vary from dullness, fever, dilated pupil to staggering gait, paralysis, epilepsy and coma.

Epilepsy

It is a sudden disturbance of cerebral function accompanied by loss of conciousness, with or without convulsion.

There is a disturbance in the functioning of the brain and causes are often related to parasites, an injury or a tumor. Signs of fits include frothing at the mouth, chattering its jaws and paddling with paws. Feces and urine are often passed involuntarily. After few minutes, the animal will quieten, lying still as if exhausted and then shortly get to its feet as if nothing had happened.

Musculoskeletal Disorders

Limping

The cat drags its leg or finds it difficult to put its full weight on it. Possible causes could be bone infection, fracture, sprain, wound, accidental injury, and tumor.

Arthritis

It is the inflammation of joints and an elderly cat may develop lameness due to the degeneration of a joint.

Skin and Coat Problems

Flea Infestation

A cat can become infested with feline, dog or human fleas, the presence of which makes the cat scratch, twitch or lick it. Fleas may carry tapeworm larvae, and can also spread some viral diseases.

Lice Infestation

The most common site is on the head, but they can make their home anywhere on the body. A heavily infested cat can become anemic.

Mite Infestation

These mites burrow into a cat's skin, causing chronic inflammation, hair loss and irritation. These affect the head and ear area producing baldness, scruffiness and dermatitis.

Fungal Dermatitis

The skin takes the form of small, circular areas with bald centers and weeping or crusty outer edges of scaly powdery skin.

Worms

The two main types of worms found in the cats are roundworms and tapeworms. Flatworms rarely infect cats in tropical areas.

Roundworms

- ☆ *Toxocara catii* – they soak up the predigested food.
- ☆ *Uncinaria* (hookworm) and *Trichuris* (whipworm) – suck the cat's blood.

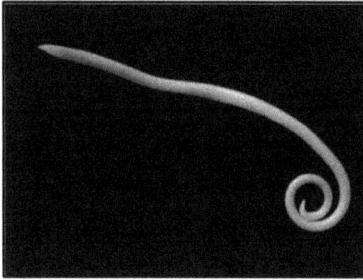

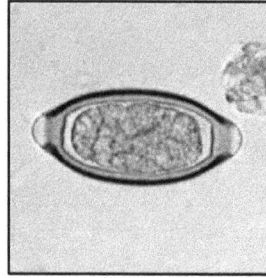

Whipworm

- ☆ Lungworm and tracheal worms – spend their life in a cat's lungs
- ☆ Heart worm

Tapeworm

- ☆ The most common tapeworm is *Dipylidium caninum*. Tapeworm infestation is easier to spot as the eggs are laid in the packages. They are moist and sticky; they also squirm and move like living things. These segments may be rectangular or cucumber like shaped.

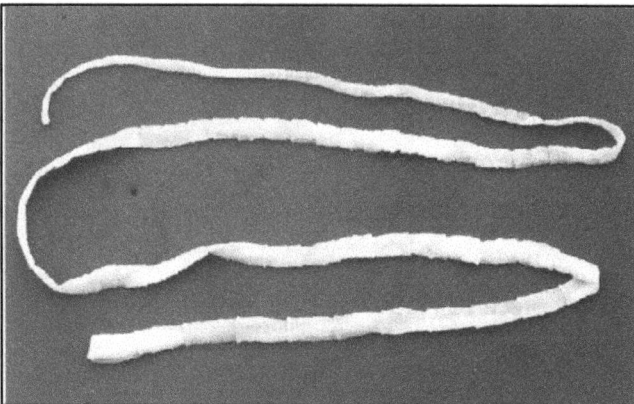

Dipylidium caninum

Chapter 33
First Aid

A Basic First Aid Kit

☆ Cotton

☆ Bandages – 4", 6"

☆ Tape Muzzle

☆ Antiseptic solution – Liquid Betadine, Savlon, etc.

☆ Antiseptic cream – Betadine, Soframycin, etc.

☆ Tweezers

☆ Scissors

☆ Thermometer

☆ Adhesive dressing

☆ Gauze

☆ A piece of cloth

☆ Q-tips

☆ Adhesive tape.

Collapse and Accident

An injured cat may need first aid action – stopping bleeding, treating shock, clearing its airways and giving artificial respiration.

Do's

1. Restrain the cat firstly in a quiet place and cover it with a blanket.
2. Check the pulse.
3. Check breathing. If irregular or nonexistent, then loosen the collar, open the mouth, pull the tongue forward, wipe away any saliva, blood or vomit and give artificial respiration.
4. Check for heartbeat.
5. Treat bleeding.
6. Look for broken bones.
7. Treat shock.
8. Contact Vet.

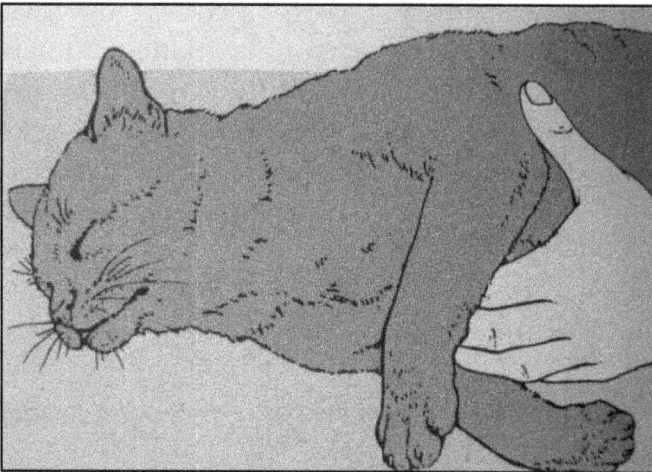

Check Heart Beet

Do Not

1. Do not move the animal unless it is in danger.

2. Do not raise its head or prop it up because saliva, blood or vomit may block the airway.

3. Do not feed animal.

Convulsions

☆ Contact the Vet immediately.

☆ Make sure that the cat is in a safe place.

☆ Leave cat where it is.

☆ Reduce external stimuli.

☆ Once fit is over, wipe the froth from the cat's mouth and clean up any urine and feces.

☆ Keep the animal indoors in quiet place until the Vet arrives.

Poisons

Cats are at risk from a number of poisons, ingested in two main ways: firstly, if a cat's coat becomes contaminated with a chemical it will lick it off in an attempt to clean itself, and secondly a cat may eat poisons used to kill pests. Don't try to make an accurate diagnosis and contact the Vet immediately.

Action

☆ Contact the Vet

☆ Wash the cat at once. Rinse it well and dry it thoroughly.

☆ Visit the Vet if you suspect a particular chemical.

Wounds and Burns

The most common cause of wounds are bites or scratches from other cats.

Action

- ☆ Clean the area
- ☆ Treat shock
- ☆ Control any bleeding
- ☆ Contact the Vet.

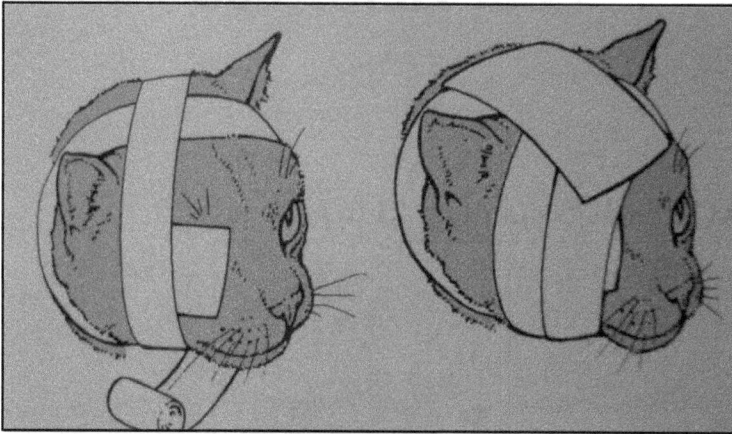

Bandaging the Eye

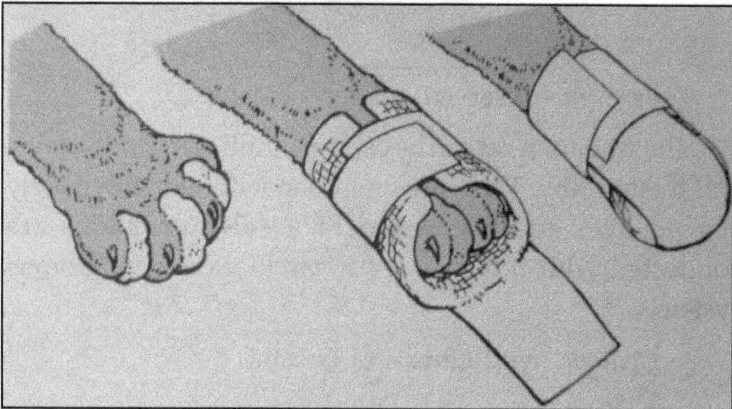

Bandaging the Injured Paw

Chapter 34
Cat Horoscope

AQUARIUS - January 21 to February 19

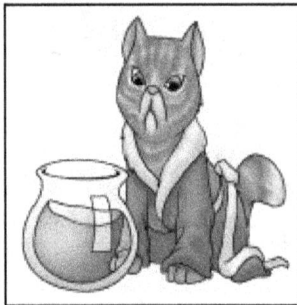

Water sign – reserved, tolerant, idealistic.

The Aquarian cat can be caring, intuitive, friendly, loyal and trustworthy. These are often slender build with widely spaced eyes and pointed ears. Health problems are connected with the legs, teeth, circulation and nervous system.

Compatible signs: Libra and Gemini

PISCES - February 20 to March 20

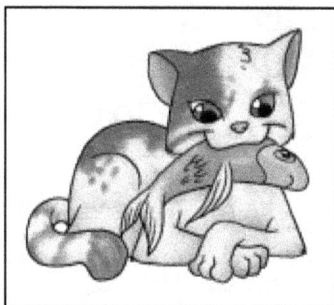

The sign of fish – imaginative, peace loving, kind.

The dreamy Piscean cat is an idealist and will exist in a fantasy world of its own. These delightful creatures are full of understanding and forgiveness. The Piscean cat often takes to water quite easily. Pisces rules the feet, liver and circulation.

Compatible signs: Cancer and Scorpio

ARIES – March 21 to April 20

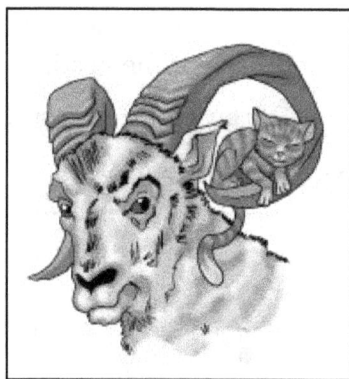

The sign of Ram – energy, leadership

The Arian cat is full of energy, and has a quick, darting appearance. They are lean, wiry and have a long slender neck. Health problems are connected with the head, brain and upper jaw.

Compatible signs: Leo and Sagittarius

TAURUS – April 21 to May 21

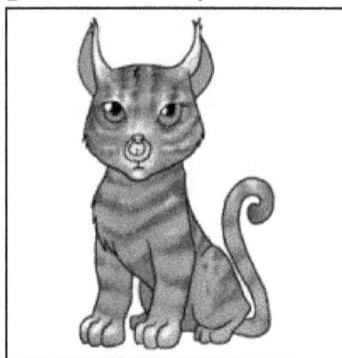

The sign of the Bull – firm, courageous and steadfast

The Taurean cat is more territorially minded than others. Positive traits include compassion, trustworthiness and practicality. Negative traits are jealousy, possessiveness and self-indulgence. Most vulnerable parts of the body are neck, throat, ears and back of the head.

Compatible signs: Virgo and Capricorn.

GEMINI – May 22 to June 21

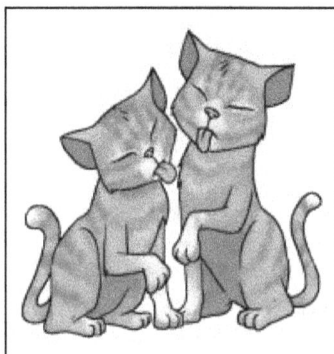

The sign of twins – duality, the intellect, versality

The Geminian cat is exuberant, energetic, versatile, adaptable, gracious and charming. Sometimes the Geminian cat can be puzzling and can cause chaos with its restless romping around the home. Health problems are related with legs, shoulders and lungs.

Compatible signs: Libra and Aquarius

CANCER – June 22 to July 23

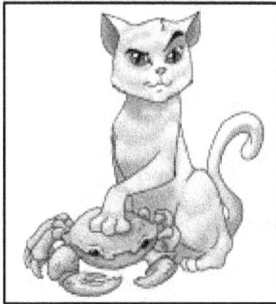

The sign of the crab – sensitive, maternal, romantic

The Cancerian cats are highly domesticated and dedicated home loving. These are often over-sensitive and vulnerable to the negative effects of dis-harmony. They are generally plump and cuddly with moon like face. These cats are prone to digestive problems.

Compatible signs: Pisces and Scorpio

LEO – July 24 to August 23

The sign of the lion – self-confidence, pride, enthusiasm

These cats are flamboyant, big-hearted and with strong sense of dignity. They demands lots and lots of attention and the Leo traits can often become negative to produce a vain, arrogant and domineering cat. Leo cats sport brilliant colors of the Sun. They usually make excellent parents and

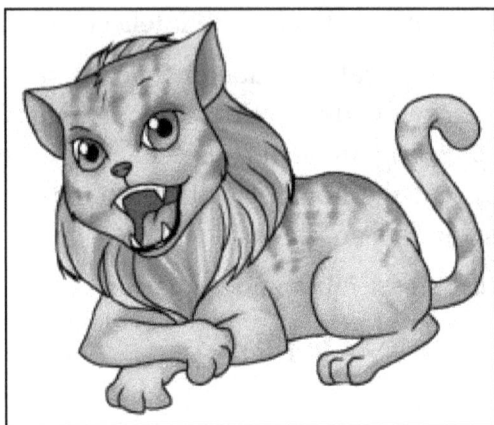

always repay the love and attention received from its owner. These cats are regal, bold and fearless. Its eyes are large, bright and impress with authoritative gaze. These are prone to heart and circulatory problems.

Compatible signs: Aries and Sagitarius

VIRGO – August 24 to September 23

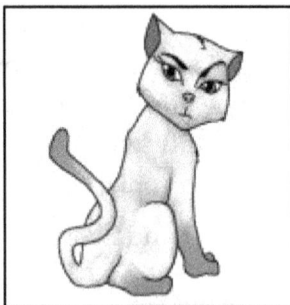

The sign of the Virgin – logical, methodical, discriminative

The Virgo cat is really cool, who is not demonstrative, likes her own space and exhibits fastidiousness regarding its health and hygiene. It is an independent cat who appreciates delicately prepared and regular meals. Bowls, intestine and abdomen are prone to the infections.

Compatible signs: Capricorn and Taurus

LIBRA – September 24 to October 23

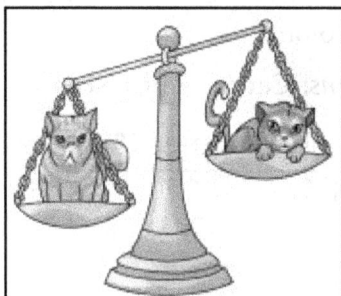

The sign of the scales – balance, love of beauty, justice

The Libran cat is intelligent, charming, lover of harmony and peace, a fine and sensitive companion. Libran cats are slender with graceful proportions. The Libran cat is prone to kidney diseases, diabetic conditions and skin complaint such as eczema.

Compatible signs: Aquarius and Gemini

SCORPIO – October 24 to November 22

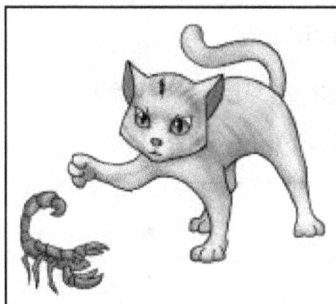

The sign of the Scorpion – tenacious, secretive, intensely psychic

The Scorpion cat has boundless energy, great strength of purpose and motivated by depth of its passion. These are great manipulators, heavy muscular and strong boned. These cats are both cautious and courageous. Negative side is jealous and vindictive. Scorpio rules the genital organs, the bladder and colon.

Compatible signs: Cancer and Pisces

SAGITARIUS – November 23 to December 21

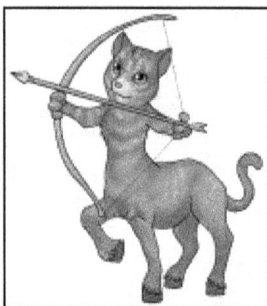

The sign of the archer – optimistic, extrovert, independent

The Sagittarian cat is a happy-go-lucky, sporty and with a well developed sense of adventure. These are an excellent mouser and are of athletic build with large, expressive eyes; love to be the centre of attention. These are more prone to accidents.

Compatible signs: Aries and Leo

CAPRICORN – December 22 to January 20

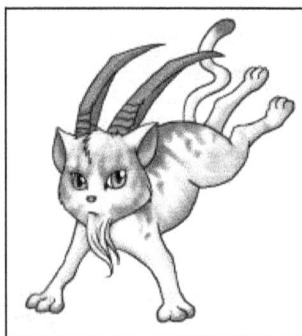

The sign of the Goat – industrious, meticulous, preserving

These are quite and self-disciplined cats. The Capricorn cat is loyal and steadfast companion. These are long-bodied and with a straight nose in an angular face, problems affecting this sign are rheumatism, cramp and a tendency to the dislocation of bones. Skin complaints such as eczema are common.

Compatible signs: Taurus and Virgo

Chapter 35
Alternative Therapy

These types of therapy should be administered by a qualified Veterinarian, or a well trained person. Physiotherapy has been widely applied in the last few years, and its benefits are well understood. Acupuncture is also quite widely prescribed, though its application is still the subject of active research.

There are many modalities included in the fields of complementary and alternative medicine.

These include:

☆ Acupuncture

☆ Homeopathy

☆ Nutraceutical therapy, supplements, vitamins and trace minerals

☆ Herbal medicine

☆ Bach flower remedies

☆ Aromatherapy

☆ Massage therapy

☆ Magnetic therapy

☆ Physiotherapy

A holistic practitioner approaches the animal as a whole and evaluates the animal's entire situation when treating the animal and his/her disease. This includes diet, environment, exercise, stress, disease symptoms, and other entities. The practitioner may use a combination of the alternative and complementary medicines listed above in addition to conventional western medicine. The goal of holistic practice is to detect and prevent disease, enhance wellness, and not just fight disease.

A brief look at some of these alternative and complementary medicines:

Acupuncture

Veterinary acupuncture has been used in China for over 3,500 years. It is the stimulation of specific points on the surface of the body most commonly by inserting thin, sterilized stainless steel needles. Acupuncture points can be stimulated by heating the point by electrical stimulation, by injecting a solution into the point, and more recently by low power laser stimulation.

Homeopathy

Homoeopathy is a complex mode of therapy and means "treat with a similar disease." Its central principle is "like cures like." The symptoms of the sick animals are matched to the remedy or remedies. The remedies are made from plants, minerals, and animal substances. Homeopathy may be used to treat acute and chronic diseases in cats such as allergies, skin conditions including feline baldness, gastrointestinal problems, cancer, and respiratory system problems such as feline asthma, among others.

First-Aid Homeopathic Medicines

☆ *Aconitum*: for fear and shock, so useful after most injuries.

☆ *Arnica*: Arnica is homeopathy's great injury remedy. Its use will minimise pain and bruising and will speed healing.

☆ *Belladonna*: High fevers with head, ear, throat or eye pain

☆ *Bryonia*: Arthritis, rheumatism, pneumonia

☆ *Calendula*: Used as a lotion, this remedy speeds healing of cuts, or open wounds

☆ *Carbo veg.*: It has ability to help patients in collapse.

☆ *Chamomilla*: Teething troubles

☆ *Hepar sulph.*: It helps patients to fight septic, purulent infections.

☆ *Hypericum*: Snakebites.

☆ *Ledum*: Wasp stings.

☆ *Nux vomica*: It helps in recovery from the intoxication.

☆ *Rhus tox.*: Rheumatism and arthritis, that are worse for first movement

☆ *Ruta*: Ligaments, tendons and other fibrous tissues are the main areas of benefit of this remedy.

☆ *Silica*: Helps the body to drive out foreign bodies, *e.g.* grass seeds.

☆ *Urtica*: Urticaria.

All of the above can be extremely useful. However, do not take any risks; if in any doubt, always consult a vet.

Nutritional Therapy, Nutritional Supplements, and Vitamins

Many problems can be cured with proper nutrition, nutritional supplements, and vitamins. Proper diet and natural supplements can support the immune system and help treat your cat's diseases. The vitamins and supplements are numerous, but vitamins A, C, and E; glucosamine; chondroitin; bioflavonoid antioxidants and certain minerals are also very helpful.

Herbal Medicine

Herbs may be helpful in the treatment of heart and circulatory problems, muscle, bone and joint conditions, behaviour problems, digestive conditions, skin diseases, and immune system problems.

Bach Flower Remedies

These are not homeopathic, herbal, or aromatic in preparation. Many other modalities of alternative and complementary medicines are becoming popular. Be sure to consult with your Veterinarian for a referral to a practitioner trained in alternative and complementary medicine.

Physiotherapy

Physiotherapy helps in restoring movement and helps facilitate your pet's body's own healing ability. This can be used to treat following conditions:

☆ Arthritis

☆ Behavioural problems

☆ Gait abnormalities

☆ Lameness

☆ Musculo-skeletal Pain

☆ Muscle imbalance

☆ Muscle weakness

☆ Muscle/Tendon/Ligament Damage

☆ Nerve Injuries

☆ Soft tissue Injuries

☆ Sports Injuries/Trauma.

Chapter 36
Cat Breeds

Persians

The Persian is well known for its temperament as well as for its beauty. They are wonderful family pets as they adapt so easily to their environment. These cats have a sturdy and rounded body with a round face and head, short and

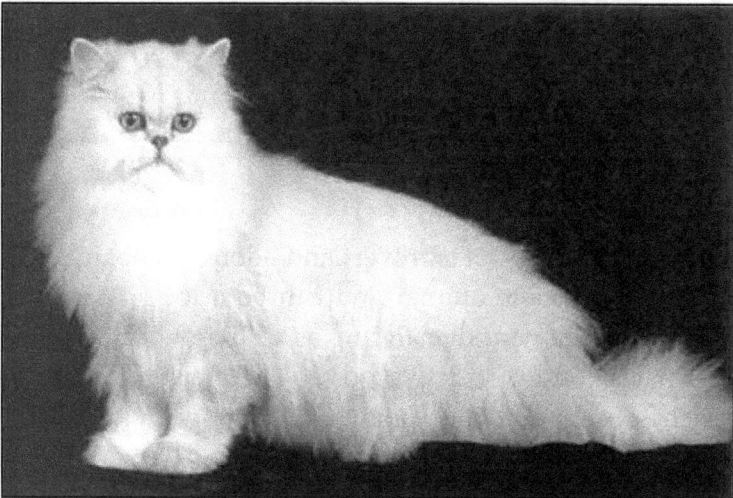

thick legs, a short nose and large, round eyes. Persians have double coat as it consists two types of hair – long, soft, woolly and slightly longer, coarser guard hairs.

Ragdoll

Ragdolls are bred in three coat patterns: Bi-color, Colorpoint and Mitted. The head is wedge-shaped with full cheeks and a short nose, slanted eye which are blue in color. The fur is long and full.

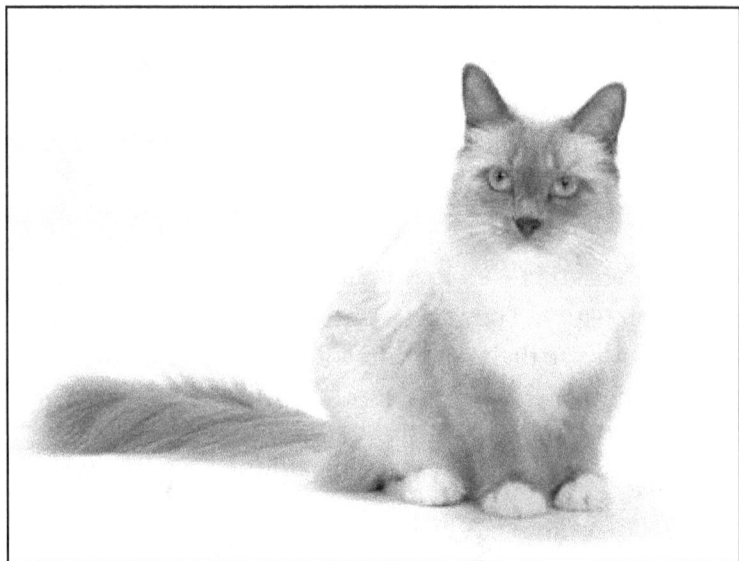

Siamese

The Siamese is an extrovert and adores company. It is very a affectionate animal and can be a loyal friend. A Siamese can be very demanding as well and can be noisy as it has a loud distinctive voice. There are four classic varieties: Seal-point, Blue-point, Chocolate-point and Lilac-point.

Bombay

Bombay coat is jet black, with a distinctive sheen, and is very short and close-lying, giving the appearance of patent leather. The Bombay has a marvellous nature and it rarely stops purring. It craves for companionship, and therefore should not be left alone for longer periods.

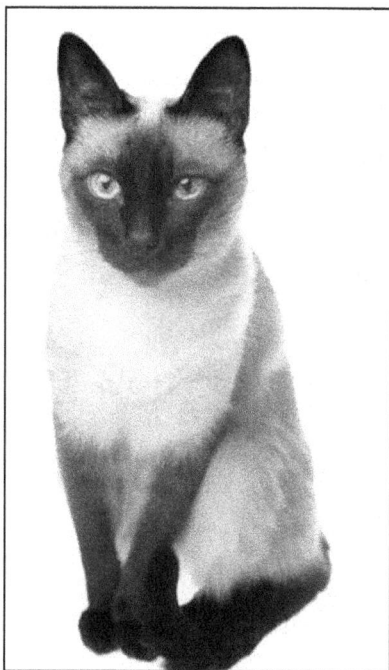

Siamese

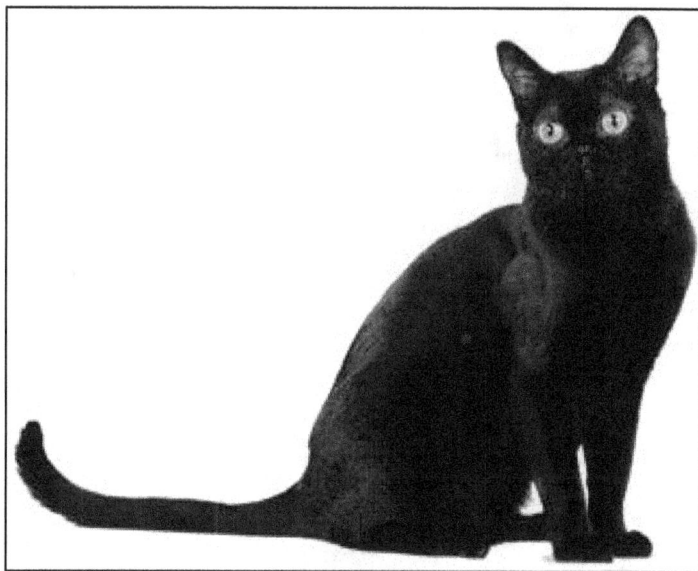

Bombay

Rex

Rex is an energetic, very affectionate and mischievous animal. The fur should be very fine and short, curlier, coarser and thinner. Body is slim type with a long tail.

Sphynx

The Sphynx is a quiet, affectionate cat and doesn't like being cuddled. A Sphynx's body feels warm to the touch, and should be taut and wrinkle free. The paws are small and rounded.

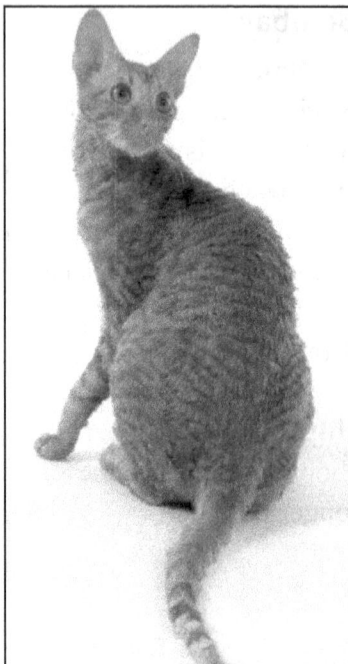

Rex

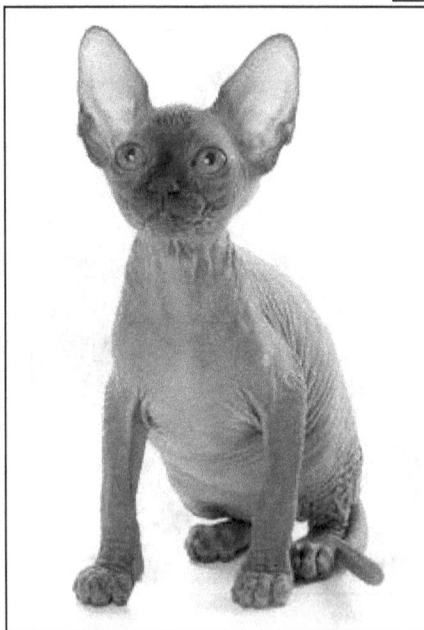

Sphynx

Index

A

Accidents, 169
Alternate therapy, 180
Anatomy, 88-94

B

Bathing, 63
Bed, 29
Boarding, 96
Bombay, 187
Breeding, 139
Breeds, 185
Brushing, 61
Burns, 171

C

Carrying cage, 28
Car travelling, 102
Coat, 59
Constipation, 132, 136
Convulsion, 170

D

Deafness, 147
Diarrhoea, 160
Disorders, 159

E

Ears, 68-72
Eggs, 167
Eyes, 66-67

F

Feeding, 144
First aid, 168
Fish, 85
Fleas, 166
Food, 55

G

Grass, 86
Grooming, 61

H

Hairball, 2, 77, 160

Health, 14, 121
Hearing, 92, 147
Horoscope, 172
Housebreaking, 43

I
Illness, 157
Indigestion, 142
Insurance, 121

K
Kittens, 20
Kneading, 90
Kennel, 96

L
Lameness, 135
Longhair, 62

M
Meat, 84
Medicines, 53-58
Milk, 148

N
Nails, 79
Name, 41, 123
Neutering, 153
Nose, 57
Nursing, 145

O
Old cat, 128
Outdoor, 105

P
Persian, 2
Play, 110
Pneumonia, 159

Poisoning, 170
Purebred, 5

Q
Quarantine, 104

R
Rabies, 115
Ragdoll, 186
Rex, 188
Ringworm, 166

S
Scratches, 79
Shelter, 7-13
Shipping, 103
Siamese, 187
Skin, 94
Sleep, 113
Smell, 92
Spay, 151
Sphynx, 188
Straying, 153

T
Tapeworms, 167
Teeth, 73
Temperature, 150
Tongue, 92
Travelling, 100

V
Vaccine, 115
Veterinarian, 124

W
Water, 87
Whiskers, 92
Worms, 166